HEAR NO EVIL

HEAR NO EVIL

Sarah Smith

TWO
ROADS

First published in Great Britain in 2022 by Two Roads
An Imprint of John Murray Press
An Hachette UK company

1

A CIP catalogue record for this title is available from the British Library

Hardback ISBN 9781529369090
Trade Paperback ISBN 9781529369106
eBook ISBN 9781529369120

Typeset in Plantin Light by
Palimpsest Book Production Ltd, Falkirk, Stirlingshire

Printed and bound in Great Britain by Clays Ltd, Elcograf S.p.A.

John Murray policy is to use papers that are natural, renewable and
recyclable products and made from wood grown in sustainable forests.
The logging and manufacturing processes are expected to conform
to the environmental regulations of the country of origin.

Two Roads
Carmelite House
50 Victoria Embankment
London EC4Y 0DZ

www.tworoadsbooks.com

In memory of my dad, John Brown, 1944-2006

'yet you want not speeche; who have your whole body for a tongue'

John Bulwer, Philocophus, 1648

∽ Thursday, 27 February 1817:
The Tolbooth Prison, Edinburgh ∽

Robert Kinniburgh climbed the High Street wearing his smartest clothes. He had been called upon by a clerk dispatched from the chambers of Lord Succoth, prominent judge and former head of judiciary. The clerk wore a pinched look and had little capacity for niceties. He waited outside the house while Robert informed a servant of his purpose, gathered his pen and notebook and pulled on his greatcoat.

Once they had reached their destination, the clerk relinquished his charge to the keeper of the Castle Street Tolbooth, Thomas Sibbald, and scurried back to his duties. Robert was shown to Jean Campbell's prison cell. It had been a cold February, yet Robert found that he was sweating under his woollen coat.

Sibbald, a gruff, heavyset man, said little as he led Robert up a narrow central staircase to a landing that fanned out in a circle and was punctuated by dark wooden doors. Each of these doors was furnished with a slit at eye level. Robert noticed that the keeper passed them without bothering to look inside. Whether Sibbald was supremely confident about the state of the people in the cells or whether there were currently no other inhabitants apart from the newly arrived Glaswegian murderess, Robert couldn't tell.

The prison itself was in a state of dilapidation. A modern facility was in the process of being built at Calton Hill and the expectation was that the Tolbooth would be demolished once the new prison was opened.

'Here we are, Mr Kinniburgh, sir,' said Sibbald, as he halted at the fifth door they came to.

The keeper raised his hand and pushed back an errant strand of thinning hair, slid a large key into the lock and turned it twice. As the door opened, Robert was struck by a cloying, sickly smell of urine and excrement but determinedly hid his disgust.

Jean Campbell was sitting on a three-legged stool on the far side of the room. She looked up at both men with a steady gaze, her demeanour calm and quiet. The cell was an odd triangular shape. Lying between the central staircase they had just climbed and the outer wall of the round tower of the Tolbooth, it made Robert think of a chunk of Stilton extracted from the cheesemonger's wheel.

He regarded the woman opposite him. This prisoner he had been summoned to interrogate. She looked thin, her body swamped in too-large prison clothes. Her dark blond hair was scraped upwards and fastened in a loose bun. She had large eyes set above deep hollows and wide cheekbones. Her pallor could be explained by her current circumstances, but Robert had been expecting to see a dead-eyed criminal of the lowest class, yet here was a woman with an intelligent expression and admirable composure.

Sibbald cleared his throat.

'This is Jean Campbell, sir.'

Robert nodded at the prisoner.

'How is the lady, Mr Sibbald?'

'She's been no trouble, sir,' the keeper replied. 'No trouble at all. I'm not sure though, sir . . .'

'Yes?'

'Forgive me, but I'm not sure how your visit will affect her. I know why you've been called in, but until now she's

2

been beyond reach and still in ignorance of the facts of the matter, so to speak.'

'Hopefully I can explain things to her,' said Robert. 'It's important she understands her situation and can give a statement of some sort to the powers that be. That way, decisions can be made on how best to deal with her.'

Sibbald nodded.

'I'm advised that she has been charged with the murder of an infant, Mr Sibbald. Do you know if it was her own child or that of someone else?'

Sibbald cast his eyes downwards. 'I believe the baby was hers, sir.'

'A tragedy,' said Robert, 'whatever the circumstances.'

'Aye. She doesn't give much away, that one, but I've heard her weeping on more than one occasion since she arrived from Glasgow. Whatever the ins and outs of the case, the lassie's broken-hairted about it.'

The keeper turned to leave them but, as he reached the door, his prisoner became agitated and let out a strange sound, like a gasp or a screech, her voice discordant. She looked at Robert and shrank into herself. Sibbald turned and approached her. He crouched down on his hunkers in front of her and took Jean's hands in his, patting them as one might a child's.

'Don't upset yourself, my dear, this is Mr Kinniburgh. I told you he was coming to see you. He's here to help you, Jean.'

Robert smiled at them both, reassuringly, he hoped. It seemed such a strange scene in this place of incarceration, torture and execution. The captive and her jailor, both occupying a much lower status in life than the well-to-do and educated visitor but both capable, nonetheless, of tender feelings and compassion.

Robert addressed the keeper.

3

'You've been able to communicate with her, Mr Sibbald?'

Sibbald looked up at him.

'Only in a very rudimentary way, sir. She seems to read my lips and understand wee bits of what I'm saying. I gesture with my hands too. Not in any proper sense, such as you might, sir. Only basic shapes and signals either of my own invention or what I've seen Jean do herself.'

At this, Jean tugged on Sibbald's sleeve to attract his attention and looked questioningly between the two men. Sibbald pointed at Robert and patted his heart. He then curled his right fist over his outstretched left palm and moved it from Robert towards Jean.

'He wants to help you. He wants to hear your story.'

At length, Jean nodded at the keeper, and did not protest when he beckoned Robert to come closer. Sibbald, meanwhile, stepped away and leant against the window frame.

Robert pulled a chair from a small table and set it down opposite Jean. She reached over to him, laying her hand on his knee. She stared at his face and then, with her thumb, she smoothed his eyebrow and trailed her fingers down his cheek. She leant back again, still watching him intently.

Robert was surprised to find himself disconcerted by the touch of the deaf woman. As a teacher at the Deaf and Dumb Institution, he spent his days with deaf children and was used to the direct way they had of communicating with him. The pupils in his care were generally more tactile than other children of his acquaintance and he had grown used to unbidden hands tapping his elbow or tugging at his clothing to get his attention. Often, his pupils would use him as a physical canvas on which to illustrate their thinking, tracing the route of a journey on his palm or describing a person by pointing at similarities or differences

4

in their teacher's appearance. Robert prided himself on adopting a fairly relaxed attitude to the personal questions that were sometimes posed to him and often disrespectful nicknames given to the staff by their charges. Jean Campbell, on the other hand, bore the marks of her current predicament and came from a class of people he didn't normally consort with but, on closer inspection, she was an attractive woman of around thirty years, not that much younger than Robert himself, and he found he was more than slightly discomfited by the way her touch made him feel.

Robert regained his composure somewhat and focused on Jean, wondering how best to indicate to her who he was and what he was there for. He felt it was important to keep things as simple as possible.

My name, he signed, pointing his index and middle fingers to his temple, and finger-spelled *ROBERT*.

Jean watched him. She began to copy the shapes of the letters but got lost halfway through. Robert repeated himself. She tried a second time but lost the thread again. As if I am offering her an exotic new concept, thought Robert. She has no alphabet.

My name, he signed, and she smiled in recognition as he tapped two fingers to his temple and pivoted them forward. Pointing back at him, she indicated her understanding.

He lip-spoke his name to her and she nodded, then drew her fingers down her cheek in an approximation of the way she had touched his face earlier.

Your name, she signed and repeated the gesture.

'The clean-shaven one.' Sibbald laughed. 'She won't have seen many of those where she comes from, sir!'

Robert looked at the stubble on Sibbald's face, his unkempt, thinning hair and spidery brows. There was no mirror in the cell, but Robert realised that, although he was not a vain man by any means, he was almost dandified in comparison with this environment and its inhabitants.

'I suppose not, Mr Sibbald.'

Robert took notice of what had just happened with Jean. This had been the most basic of exchanges and yet it had told him so much. He shifted in his seat and began to communicate with her, using limited signs and reinforcing important information with a combination of repetition, lip-speaking and nodding, in the hope that it would help her to follow him.

Lord Succoth's note had contained a brief explanation to the effect that the court wished to discover if Jean was fit to plead in any practical or meaningful sense. The authorities were required to make a considered judgement about whether Jean could answer questions put to her by both the prosecution and defence advocates in a court of law and whether she was able, morally and intellectually, to understand what she had done and what the consequences of her actions might be.

If she stood trial, it would be the first time a deaf person had been examined in a Scottish court. If she was found guilty of murder, she was likely to be hanged. Robert couldn't help but wonder what Lord Succoth imagined might be his part in that turn of events.

Robert and Jean faced one another. The system he had settled on for the moment was crude and hardly sufficient for the task entrusted to him but, for now, it would have to do. It was all they had.

~ Friday, 28 February 1817:
Chessels Court, Edinburgh ~

Robert watched his wife at the stove as she spooned globules of batter onto an iron girdle and piled the results on a large serving dish. They looked for all the world like a tower of pebbles on the sands at Portobello.

Margaret turned to him, spatula in hand. 'Tell me then,' she asked, 'what are we to do today? Without you.'

'I've written some instructions,' Robert replied, holding up a piece of paper. 'You and Isabella can see to the girls and I've made out a list of lessons for the boys. Joseph can take the lead. Just keep an eye on them, for me, will you? Make sure none of the lads take my absence as a cue for dawdling?'

'I'm sure we'll muddle through,' said Margaret.

Robert smiled, refusing to rise to her pointed tone. 'I've no doubt you'll do better than muddle through.'

He sat down at the long kitchen table and spread butter over a still-warm drop-scone and ate it quickly, burning the inside of his mouth.

They were both up earlier than usual. Robert, because he was due back at the Tolbooth first thing and had been instructed to call in to Lord Succoth's chambers on his way. He was expected to report on his initial meeting with Jean Campbell and to give His Lordship some idea of what progress might be expected in the case now that they had a potential interpreter on hand.

Margaret had woken at the same hour as her husband and, rather than turn over and go back to sleep, she had decided to steal a march on the day by making a start on preparing breakfast for the pupils. Usually, she and Robert rose at the same time as Margaret's sister, Isabella, and two of the older female pupils. The women seeing to cooking and laying tables, Robert enjoying a short spell in his private office before another school day's labours began.

There was a curious and unexpected intimacy to their being left to themselves, in the kitchen, while the rest of the household slept on. They lay in bed together every night and were private and close there, but whereas other couples of their status might share their dwelling with a housekeeper or a maid-of-all-work, the Kinniburghs navigated their way through a small army of staff, relatives and pupils and were rarely alone together.

Margaret brought a pot of tea to the table, along with two cups and a jug of milk, and sat down alongside him. She poured the tea and handed him a cup. She took his knife and cut a buttered dropped scone in half, helping herself to one of the pieces. She pushed it greedily into her mouth and smiled at him.

'What's she like, your murderess?' Margaret swallowed and widened her eyes in mock sensation.

Robert frowned.

'She's not necessarily guilty, Maggie.'

Margaret gave a theatrical sigh and raised her hands in a pleading gesture. 'I know, I know, but I want an exciting story from you. You were so distracted last night that I hardly got a peep out of you.'

'It's not a tale in a book, you know,' Robert said. 'She's a real person who may have to face the fatal consequences of what she's been accused of. Courts don't tend to look kindly on infanticide.'

8

'I don't mean to make light of her predicament,' said Margaret, reaching out and touching his arm. 'I can be serious. It might help to talk about it. What has she told you so far? Has she admitted to killing the baby?'

Robert shook his head. 'No, she hasn't. It's sometimes difficult to follow what she's trying to say. It took most of yesterday to get an idea of how I might speak with her and discover some of her background. It would have helped if I had been properly briefed instead of wheeched away up to the prison without being given the full facts of the case.'

Robert rolled his tongue over the burn inside his mouth. It felt raw, sore and oddly comforting.

'How did you communicate with her?' Margaret asked. 'Does she use signs?'

'Some,' said Robert. 'She appeared to lip-read a great deal, but she recognised a few of the more common-place signs I used; gestures for name and place, for example. Some of the signs she used were unfamiliar to me, but that could simply be that they're local to her own place.'

'Can she read and write at all?'

Robert shook his head.

'What do the courts expect you to do with her?'

'To find out if she can communicate or be communi-cated to,' Robert said. 'At least, well enough for the various legal processes to take place.'

Margaret regarded her husband for a moment.

'They will leave it to you to make the decision?' she asked.

'I suppose they will,' said Robert.

'It seems a very great burden.'

Robert frowned. 'You think it beyond me?'

Margaret reached out and took his hand, laced her fingers

in his. 'I don't doubt that you can make an assessment of this woman's faculties, Robbie. It's just that I wonder what the extent of your involvement in the case is likely to be.'

'What do you mean?'

'If you tell Lord Succoth that Jean Campbell can communicate, then she'll need you to relay any testimony she gives. Quite apart from the responsibility, it could prove time consuming. If you are unsure, you shouldn't make any claims on her behalf.'

Robert took his hand from hers, lifted his cup and took a drink. The clerk who had collected him yesterday had indicated that he would be paid a sizeable hourly rate for his time. If called to trial, he would be afforded the status of an expert witness and remunerated appropriately. Any extra monies would benefit the school and compensate for his absence.

'I think it's important work, Maggie.'

Margaret gave a tight smile and stared at the damp tealeaves that patterned the bottom of her cup. 'What is it like, inside the Tolbooth?' she asked, puncturing the silence between them.

Robert followed her lead. 'Empty and incredibly cold. I think Jean Campbell is their only prisoner. I don't know how Sibbald stands it. It feels like a place that has had all of its energy and usefulness leached out of it.'

'Mr Sibbald, is he the jailor? Does he pace up and down rattling his keys?'

Robert laughed. 'Not that I noticed. He's quite ordinary really and surprisingly thoughtful regarding his prisoner.'

Margaret shivered. 'To be shut away like that. The poor woman. No matter what she's done, I wouldn't wish that on my worst enemy.'

'There has to be justice, Maggie. We must answer for our actions.'

'I suppose so, but to be deaf and alone in there. Not able to understand what strangers are saying to you. She must be very frightened.'

Robert considered this for a second. 'She doesn't seem frightened. Unhappy to be imprisoned. Frustrated perhaps, but she shows no fear. It's as if she has complete confidence in her professed innocence.'

'But she threw her baby into the Clyde, Robbie. How can she be innocent of that?'

'I have no idea. I suppose that's what I need to try to determine. If I could get her to tell me the whole story, I might have a chance, but I don't know how to persuade her to trust me. For all she knows, I might be in the pay of those who wish to do her harm.'

As they spoke, familiar noises began to reverberate around the building. Footsteps upstairs and the opening and closing of doors. The household readying itself for the day. Margaret rose from the table and began clearing away their breakfast dishes.

She bent down and kissed the top of his head.

'What are you so worried about? They wouldn't have called you in if they didn't think you'd be able to help,' she said, gently.

'Succoth will want answers straight away.'

Margaret shrugged. 'Well, he'll just have to wait, won't he? Why would she immediately tell her story to you? That's not the way deaf people are with the hearing. You should know that.'

Robert laughed in spite of himself. 'I don't think Lord Succoth will be much concerned with the intricacies of the deaf world, do you?'

'I suppose not,' Margaret conceded. 'But he can hardly

expect you to provide a coherent story when you've only just met the woman and have nothing to offer her to give her hope.'

~ Friday, 28 February 1817:
Adam Square, Edinburgh ~

Robert buttoned up his tailcoat, lifted his hat, and left the
Deaf and Dumb Institution by the kitchen entrance. The
trees in the back courtyard were skeletal against a bleached
morning sky. The new gardens had not had time to establish themselves and there were no spring flowers as yet to
fill the bare pockets of earth.

He let himself out by way of a rough wooden door that
led to the junction with the Cowgate and walked up
towards Lord Succoth's residence. It was only eight in
the morning, but the streets were already restless. Dust
and stour billowed from carts leaving the coal yard, the
overworked horses' breath rank and smoky in the cold
air.

Robert dodged across the street and picked his way
around the filthy, open sewers of the Cowgate, and into
the slightly more salubrious surroundings of the High
School and Infirmary. Despite the assured aspect he had
presented to Maggie, he felt some anxiety at reprising the
role of expert in front of His Lordship, and took a moment
to gather himself as he crossed the square.

Lord Succoth lived in a large townhouse at Adam Square
that was also home to his offices, and was populated by a
small staff. Robert presented himself at the business
entrance to the building and was shown to a small waiting

room by a very young man with flushed cheeks and sober dress who he presumed to be some sort of apprentice writer or junior secretary.

After a few minutes, the pinched-looking clerk from the previous day stuck his head around the door and asked Robert to follow him. Robert dutifully trotted along behind while the clerk led him through narrow corridors, the walls covered in flaked and yellowed distemper, and up a stone stairway to reach the main part of the house.

'I'm afraid Lord Succoth is still breakfasting, Mr Kinniburgh.'

The clerk had long, skinny legs that fairly scuttled along, his leather-soled shoes clattering as they met the bare floorboards.

'Oh,' said Robert, 'I was under the impression His Lordship wished to see me as early as possible this morning. Before I return to the Tolbooth.'

'Just so, just so,' asserted the clerk, over his shoulder. 'The earlier the better, in light of the task before us all. There's no time to waste. He asked that I show you upstairs as soon as you arrived.'

'Thank you,' Robert replied. 'I'm sorry, but I'm afraid I didn't catch your name yesterday.'

'No need,' the clerk declared. 'Perhaps I didn't introduce myself properly, what with the urgency of my errand.'

The clerk spun round and reached out his hand to shake Robert's own. 'It's Gibson, Archibald Gibson. Senior Writer to His Lordship.'

Gibson resumed his journey and pushed open a door at the top of the stairs. They emerged into a spacious hall painted in a dark shade of green. Light flooded in from an atrium window in its high central ceiling. An elaborate staircase curled up towards the next storey of the house and, around it, detailed, ornamental plasterwork was picked out in yellow and gold.

Gibson gestured to another door. 'Lord Succoth will see you in the morning room, sir.'

Robert followed Gibson's lead and went inside. Lord Succoth was sitting in a winged armchair that had its back to them and the clerk cleared his throat to attract his employer's attention.

'Mr Kinniburgh to see you, sir.'

Succoth rose from his seat. Robert had seen His Lordship in the streets around the High Court of Justiciary, surrounded by his official retinue. On those occasions, Succoth had been bewigged and cloaked. This morning, he was less formally dressed, but no less imposing. Despite his relatively small stature and advancing years, Lord Succoth had the lean, bronzed aspect of a former prize fighter who might still prove handy in the ring.

'Ah. Kinniburgh. Welcome. Please join me.' Succoth pointed to another seat nearby. 'Can I offer you some coffee? Or something to eat?'

'No thank you, Your Lordship, I've breakfasted already.'

Lord Succoth sipped his coffee and set it down again on the table.

'Well, Kinniburgh, how did you find our prisoner yesterday?'

Robert cleared his throat. 'Tolerably well, sir. I made some headway communicating by signs. The lady is not used to literacy and has no access to an alphabet. It was slow progress, I'm afraid.'

Succoth sniffed. 'Aye, I can't imagine she's the easiest person to interview. Dirty and stupid, I'm led to believe.'

Robert stiffened. 'She's certainly poor, sir, but I wouldn't necessarily describe her as either dirty or stupid. Reticent – certainly – but not completely unforthcoming.'

'Indeed? She's deaf and dumb, though. That's correct, isn't it?'

15

'Well, yes, Your Lordship, but that can't be used as a measurement of one's intelligence. Being deaf certainly makes it more difficult for someone to navigate their way through society, sir. In my experience, those who manage to carve out any sort of life for themselves are often much more intelligent than those born with the gift of hearing.'

Lord Succoth suppressed a laugh. 'Jean Campbell's a hoor from the Glasgow slums, Kinniburgh. Hardly some kind of noble savage.'

Robert shifted in his seat and changed the subject.

'I'm afraid I was at a disadvantage. Yesterday, I mean. I had scant information before I spoke to Jean Campbell other than what your clerk and the keeper were able to tell me.'

Succoth took another sip of coffee and then reached for his pipe. He tapped out the remnants of his last smoke into a pewter ashtray.

'She was seen to throw a baby's body from a bridge into the River Clyde,' Succoth said. 'When apprehended, the police sergeant in Glasgow sent for a local deaf man known to have a bit of speech in the hope that he might induce her to tell them what had occurred. This fellow spoke to her at length, apparently, but she is said to have simply shrunk into herself and refused to give any more details about what happened. Is that because she is deliberately withholding her story from us or that she can't understand the questions being asked of her? This is the conundrum that we wish you to answer for us, Kinniburgh.'

'I would like to help, sir, but I'm still unsure how quickly I can answer these questions for you, Your Lordship.'

Succoth opened a tin of tobacco and began to pack the worm-like strands into the chamber of his pipe with a finger. 'I'll make it financially worth your while, Kinniburgh. I assume you need funds to keep your school going?'

Robert nodded. 'Indeed.'

'Well, then. Let us work together to winkle the truth out of prisoner Campbell's shell.'

Succoth's earlier comment still rankled with Robert.

'You referred to her as a prostitute, Your Lordship. What made you say that?' he asked.

'According to the Glasgow police, she lives over the brush with a papist called Donnelly. Although that hardly narrows things down, given the preponderance of Irish infesting the west of Scotland. By all accounts, she has an older son who was born in Glasgow. Campbell herself is rumoured to hail from Argyll.'

'I would like to carry on interviewing Jean Campbell, sir,' Robert said. 'However, if I am to find out the information you require – about the crime itself and the events leading up to it – I may need some time. We have many signs in common but by no means all.'

Succoth nodded and waved away this advice. Less in dismissal, thought Robert, than in a pretence of understanding the complexities of communicating with the deaf.

'The prisoner's deafness aside,' said Robert, 'we are dealing with a woman who has lost her baby under circumstances of some violence. If she is innocent of the charge of murder, her grief must be intolerable.'

'Do not presume her innocent, Kinniburgh. I've known many a hard ticket that was able to turn on the tears when it suited.'

'I presume nothing, Your Lordship, I am merely taking into consideration my initial impressions of the task at hand.'

'Aye, well,' said Succoth, 'information is what I'm after, impressions are of no use to the law.'

Robert's instinct was to debate this point with Succoth,

who, he believed, was as guilty as anyone of making judgements based on first impressions. His head, however, cautioned him to caw canny and concentrate on the matter at hand. There was nothing to be gained by going against His Lordship at this early stage.

'I assure you, sir, my immediate concern is to establish a mode of communication to allow the prisoner's testimony to be heard.'

Succoth gave a small nod of satisfaction and sat back in his chair. 'The more detail you can get from her and the quicker you can relay it to me, Kinniburgh, the better.'

Robert nodded. 'I may find it helpful to visit Glasgow at some stage. To confirm the background to the case. Would that be acceptable?'

His Lordship pulled on his pipe and let the smoke escape from his mouth in tendrils, curling upwards. The smell of an expensive rub of tobacco hung in the air.

'Certainly, Kinniburgh. Gibson will pass on any information that you request and make travel arrangements should you require them.'

'Thank you, sir.'

Succoth stood up and Robert followed suit.

'Keep me abreast of developments, Kinniburgh.'

4

∼ Friday, 28 February 1817:
The Tolbooth Prison, Edinburgh ∼

Robert explained to Jean that she had been charged with a crime. According to witnesses, she had thrown her child into the Clyde. But, as no body had been found, it was difficult to determine if this was, in fact, the case.

Robert raised an index finger and pulled his wrists together.

When a person is arrested, he signed, *the police must hear their story.*

The police didn't understand Jean, so she needed to tell her story to him. He made a curved shape using both of his index and middle fingers.

On the bridge, what happened?

Jean shook her head violently. Anger or fear. Robert couldn't be sure. She brought her right hand up sharp and flat over her head. What is she saying, thought Robert? *I'll be dead? They'll kill me?*

He raised a pointed finger towards his brow and, with a frustrated expression, shook his head.

I don't understand. Plaintively, he curved his hand and offered it to her. *Please, I want to help you.*

Thomas Sibbald sat watching, quietly, but shifted in his chair at Jean's frantic gestures. He likely understood only a little of what passed between them, but Robert noted the man's look of concern. Most people were terrified of hanging, right enough. And Sibbald had seen his fair share of the drop. Fear could be catching. In his job, you'd learn to build up your immunity.

Jean sat still for a moment, thinking. Then she drew herself up and looked squarely in Robert's eyes.

I'm not a bad woman, she signed.

I know. I know, agreed Robert. *Tell me what happened. Why were you on the bridge?*

Jean's eyes glistened with unspent tears. *I ran for a long time. I needed to rest for a moment, get my breath back. I had to get away from him. I was frightened he would find me.*

Robert looked quizzically at Sibbald for a moment, but the keeper looked just as confused as he was, so he turned back to Jean. Robert's brow furrowed, and he formed a spiral with his index finger.

Who?

Jean began to rock rhythmically back and forth, holding tightly to the sides of her wooden chair.

I'm going too quickly, thought Robert, I'll lose her. He reached out, placing the palms of his hands onto Jean's shoulders. Trying to contain her panic, to rescue her from the onslaught of memory and bring her back to this day, to this room.

An earthenware jug perched on a nook in the wall. Sibbald rose and poured some small beer into a tumbler and handed it to Jean, his calloused hand curling her thin fingers around its cold surface. Robert moved back into his seat and both men waited patiently while she drank.

In the still of the prison cell, a tableau crept into Robert's mind. He imagined himself in the boardroom of the Deaf and Dumb Institution in Chessels Court, standing in a corner of the room while the eminent judge, Lord Succoth, mingled with board members, drinking whisky and toasting the king. Someone noticed Robert's presence and gestured towards him. The entire company shifted nervously until Lord Succoth muttered something under his breath and they all laughed. Robert tried in vain to speak to them, but they turned their backs deliberately and with impunity.

It was a fancy. Nothing of the sort had ever happened. Nevertheless, he could see the possibility that his hard-won career might slip through the cracks of the floorboards in Jean's prison cell. Robert stood up and walked to the tiny opening in the external wall of the cell. He drew on a shaft of cold, fresh air and stared down to the pan tiles on the roof below.

After a few moments, Jean appeared by his side and clutched his arm. She gestured to him, apologetically, to sit down.

Take your time. I'm in no hurry, he signed. *You talked of a man. Who did you mean?*

She steeled herself.

I was afraid that he would kill me. He had secrets.

About the baby? asked Robert.

She nodded. *He told me to keep quiet.*

And you did? You kept the secrets?

I thought no one would understand me or they wouldn't believe me.

Why would they not believe you?

He would say I was a liar, a deaf and dumb hoor.

Jean raised her arm, twirled her wrist and Robert blushed at the term and cursed his manners.

Why would he call you that name?

Jean shrugged.

I don't know. Because I'm poor? Because I'm not married?

Who? Robert signed again, exasperated. *Who is this man?*

I cannot tell you, signed Jean. *I am frightened of him. He is frightened of me. But he can hurt me more. He told me to stay silent.*

21

Jean pinched her thumb and forefinger together and gestured the locking of her lips. Her eyes were wet, and her breath stuttered in her throat.

Sibbald stood up.

'Perhaps, sir, this would be a good time to let the prisoner rest? I have a pot of tea on the hob downstairs.'

~

Jean watched the two men leave and the door close behind them, stealing the thin shaft of light they had brought in. She had only been there a few days, but she knew the cell like the back of her hand. Stone walls, straw bed, wooden chairs and a table. A pot to piss and shit in. Not much, but it was no worse than the filth of Taylor's Close or her father's tiny cottage exposed to the elements on Islay. At least here Mr Sibbald locked her in where no one could get to her. There were worse things than being caged.

5

~ Friday, 28 February 1817:
The Tolbooth Prison, Edinburgh ~

Jean crouched at the stone fireplace nestled into the wall of her cell. She picked around her fingertips, ripped at a hangnail and winced. Robert's questions had pulled her mind back to the previous week, the night her baby had been consumed by the river and the world had tipped on its axis.

When the cry had gone up near the Old Bridge, the local constable had been first on the scene, waving and winding his rattle aloft. As he bent down to scrutinise her, Jean had caught the smell of old meat on his breath.

It took some time for his colleagues to join him. In the cramped warrens off the Saltmarket, the rattles the police carried could alert watchmen and other constables but, more often than not, they ran in the opposite direction away from the trouble. That was if they ran at all, most watchmen being elderly and just as likely to be found dozing in a guard box as patrolling with their lanterns. The candles these old men were given supplemented their wages and were a valuable commodity more use to them off duty than on the job.

She couldn't hear the rattle, but Jean recognised it and knew what it meant. She was aware of much more than people gave her credit for. Always had been. Sometimes she railed against the way people decided for themselves how much she understood. Other times it suited her fine to be thought a fool. They either looked down on you or felt sorry for you. Not once did any hearing person treat her like she was the same as them. She had a language that they didn't understand.

The cell in the Tolbooth had a narrow, barred window. Jean could see the light of day or the encroaching dark of evening as a sliver of colour or a faint scent of rain or the sting of frost. Often, she noticed a flicker of seagull wings pass overhead, on their way back from plundering fish at the docks or swooping down to scavenge amongst the muck that gathered in the wynds and pends of Edinburgh. The sun's wane at twilight and the sky's plunge into inky blue signalled the oncoming night. She could reckon all of these things although she could not hear.

She walked over to the pallet bed in the far corner of the room and lay down on it. She would rest her eyes for a while, until the man with the questions came back. She wondered about him. Something in his nature made her want to lay her troubles out before him. To ask him for something, she wasn't sure what. Help, understanding, absolution?

The intensity of what she had experienced during the past weeks made it difficult to unravel her story, even to herself. She had begun with the best of intentions; to provide her child with a home and help another soul into the bargain. How had that man twisted what she had done? Distorted it into a cold-hearted transaction that he could use to threaten her and buy her silence?

Jean opened her eyes and looked up at the ceiling. The plaster was worn in places, exposing clumps of horsehair that had been left behind as it crumbled away. Her mind shifted back to this latest, kind man, who knew the signs and the ways of the deaf, even though he could hear. Could she trust herself to trust him?

~

An hour or so later, when the two men returned, Robert had decided to take a different tack.

Where do you come from? Were you born in Glasgow?
Jean shook her head.

No. From an island. Islay. Do you know where that is?
Robert nodded. He had never been to the Hebrides, but he knew that Jean's birthplace was to the south and west of the country, owned by the Campbells of Shawfield, although he doubted Jean was a scion of that eminent family. As far as he knew, Islay was a place of farming and fishing, populated by scattered groups of inhabitants who lived a life largely untouched by the scientific and philosophical advances enjoyed by the cities and towns on the mainland.

Robert motioned to Jean to elaborate.

I was born in a cottage, near Bowmore. She used her hands to suggest the playing of a fiddle.

Were you born deaf? Robert asked, raising two fingers and placing them on his ear.

Jean nodded.

In the beginning, they didn't know it, but as I got older, my mother noticed that I didn't speak like my brothers and didn't turn when she called me. But I could hear my mother, all the same.

Robert looked incredulous. *What do you mean?* he asked.

When she held me, I could feel the words at her throat and recognise the smell of the sea on her skin. Sometimes she sang. Jean pinched the thumb and forefinger of both hands together to signify music. *As she made music, I felt every rise and fall of her breast.*

Robert clenched his fist and gathered it towards his brow.

I remember the songs my own mother sang to me. That

memory is very clear. Sometimes I wonder if feelings carry further than sound.

She leant towards him across the shaft of light spilling from the narrow window.

Yes. Perhaps. Even in this place, I feel her arms wrap around me, trying to comfort me in my trouble.

Your mother loved you very much, I think, said Robert.

Jean nodded. *My mother would pat my back as a baby. Later, I began to pat her back too. I think I learnt the love that was held in that small movement.*

Thomas Sibbald shifted in his chair.

Robert looked at Jean and smiled sympathetically. She was talking more freely, and he wondered if that was because her mind was concentrated on good memories and had shifted, however briefly, from the death of her child.

Take me to the cottage. I'd like to know about your home.

Just a plain house, Jean shrugged. *Two rooms and a bit of land. We had a few cattle and my father and brothers worked on the lead mining. I was the youngest. The only girl.*

Robert smiled. *Your brothers, they would have made a great fuss of you?*

They would push and shove each other to be the first to tell me their stories. Donnie always made me laugh. He would take my mother's bonnet from its hook, her pinny from the washing line and parade up and down, pretending to be one of the old gossips from the village.

Jean turned her gaze downwards.

It was difficult to make a living from the land. But it's been harder to be away for so long.

What made you leave? Robert asked.

I met a man, and I was to have a baby. My parents feared I would meet with disgrace. So, I came to Glasgow to live with my mother's brother and his wife. Once Sandy was born, I left him with my aunt and cousins and got work.

26

Where were you able to find work? Robert asked.

A cotton mill. There was one nearby. My aunt asked around and helped me to get the job.

Sibbald had been sitting in the corner of the cell. Not able to follow what Robert and Jean were discussing, he had begun to doze off. Now he yawned. He stood up and stretched. His shirt rode up, exposing, for a moment, an expanse of mottled belly. The keeper of the Tolbooth rubbed his hands together, purposefully.

'Would you excuse me for a time, Mr Kinniburgh? I have some duties to attend to. You're welcome to stay and carry on talking with Jean. There's a bell on the landing that you can ring if you need anything.'

'Yes, of course, Mr Sibbald. I wouldn't want you to be inconvenienced any more than necessary.'

Sibbald took his leave and Robert turned his attention to Jean once more.

Sandy's father, was he not willing to marry you? Could no way be found for you to stay in your birthplace?

Jean shrugged. *He had a wife already.*

Although Jean had talked of disgrace, Robert saw no evidence of shame or remorse in her eyes. A hint of regret, perhaps? Was that for her transgression – as ought to be the case – or simply for the loss of this man? He feared for her mortal soul if she hankered after some illicit relationship rather than atoning for her sin.

Still, he was not here to judge the morals of others.

Through the narrow opening in the cell wall, he could see the gloom of the winter's afternoon beginning its descent into darkness. He had deserted his family, his school and his charges for the best part of the day. He must pursue his objective. Albeit cautiously. He didn't want Jean to falter in the way she had earlier.

Robert stretched out the thumbs and index fingers of

both hands and pointed them outwards from his mouth, like a pair of pistols.

Your family in Islay, did they speak Gaelic or English?

Everyone had the Gaelic. My mother knew some English because she had worked in service before she married. Later, when I got to Glasgow, all I understood was how she mouthed the words for cutlery and cooking.

Robert smiled. *Did you make signs on Islay?*

No. Not proper signing like they have here. We just made them up as we needed them. I'd never met another deaf person until I came to Glasgow. Jean stopped for a moment and gave this some thought. *I knew old people who had lost their hearing, but not like me. Not born deaf.*

Robert noticed that Jean signed *Glasgow* by bringing her clenched fists together and then lacing her fingers to make a shape similar to a beamed roof. These were the finger shapes that spelled out *G* and *W* and were brought together to make the sign for the city. But if he were to finger-spell a word using those letters, along with others – *wig*, for example, or *grow* – he knew she wouldn't follow his logic and connect his movements with the concept of a wig or the action of growing.

Robert recognised that, despite his years of training and working with deaf people, his own starting point for all forms of communication was textual and the alphabet was his bedrock.

Jean approached it by a different route, one which sought out the most important object to be discussed and spun out from the centre. Robert knew he must endeavour to follow her pattern, rather than rely on the linear pathways inherent in a language that could be written down.

Jean yawned as the cathedral bell tolled the hour and drew a blanket around her shoulders. It must be at least five o'clock, thought Robert. Darkness had crept around them so gradually that they had barely noticed. He gestured to a tallow candle by Jean's bed, and she leant down and passed it to him so that he could light it from the scattering of coal and ash that lay in the fireplace.

When he had handed the lighted candle back to her, he signed, *I have to go home. I will come back tomorrow. Perhaps we can talk about the people you met in Glasgow then?*

She nodded and stood up as he left the room and pulled the door shut behind him. The keeper had left the heavy key in place and Robert hesitated, unsure of what to do. He wasn't a jailor and yet he worried that Sibbald might regard him as lacking responsibility if he left the cell unlocked.

He reached down and touched the protruding iron bow. Its faint rattle made him jump. Simultaneously, he turned the key and caught sight of Jean through the slit in the thick door as she glanced round. Their eyes met and something inside him recoiled. What was it?

Robert made a fist and gripped the key as he descended the stairwell. He felt an uneasy pull both of attraction and repulsion.

6

Dusk brushed the sandstone of the square-fronted villa on Partickhill Road and softened its edges.

Charles McDougall sat in the drawing room, smoking his pipe. He was still wearing his outdoor clothes, although he had been home for at least an hour.

Upstairs, his wife, Euphemia, lay sleeping under blankets and eiderdown while a fire trembled its last in the grate.

On his arrival home, Charles had sent Martha, the house-maid, out with a letter to deliver some distance away. The house was silent, and the room darkened as the winter sun dipped from view.

Charles glanced towards the ceiling and heaved himself up. He knocked out the contents of his pipe into the fire-place and laid it on the mantelpiece. In the hallway, he took off his greatcoat and muffler and hung them on the coat stand. He climbed the stairs and let himself into Euphemia's room using a key that lay on a semi-circular table next to her bedroom door.

His wife slumbered on and Charles gathered up the waxed brown paper that had contained her sleeping draught, folded it neatly and placed it in the top drawer of a small writing bureau in front of the window. This window was an echo of the one below but, from the upper storey of the house, the view was more expansive. A broad dirt path snaked down the hill to Dumbarton Road and towards new warehouses built where the River Clyde was being widened and improved. At intervals, numerous ships' masts punctuated the darkening sky like a ribbon of sheet music winding its way to the sea.

Behind him, Euphemia twisted round onto her back and began to snore softly. He looked over at her and noticed that the top buttons of her nightdress hadn't been done up properly. Whoever had put his wife to bed earlier must have struggled to get her out of her stained dress and into her bedclothes as the sleeping draught took effect. He tried to rectify this mistake, but the starched cotton, tiny mother-of-pearl buttons and his thick fingers combined to frustrate him.

'Christ almighty,' he muttered. He made a cursory attempt at smoothing Euphemia's hair. Strands of coarse grey sprang from the brown, spitefully refusing to be tamed. Euphemia wore a plain kind of linen mobcap to bed as a rule but, in the haste of the day, no one had remembered about it. Charles's eyes swept the room, but he couldn't see it lying anywhere. Even if he had, he wouldn't have known how to put it on. What had he come to? A man of his position attending a lunatic wife.

He sat, perched on the pile of bed linen, for a few moments. Glowering, watching the shallow rise and fall of Euphemia's breath.

He leant over and whispered, 'I will never forgive you, you fucking selfish bitch.'

~

At eight o'clock in the evening, the maid returned from her errand and a bell rang from Charles's study to summon her before she had a chance to change into her house shoes and cap. She hurried upstairs feeling more than a little aggrieved but rearranged her face and knocked on the door.

'Come in,' barked Charles.

'Excuse me, sir,' said Martha, entering the room.

She cast her eyes downwards in a gesture of submission although, behind them, her mind staged a little fantasy where she bludgeoned the old swine with a poker from the fire and blamed it on a pack of papist robbers.

'Well? Did you deliver the note I gave you for Dr Wilson?'

'Yes, sir, I did, sir. Only he wasn't there himself, so I left it with his wife, who assured me she would pass it on to the doctor.'

Charles drummed his fingers on the wood of the mantelpiece.

'Did Mrs Wilson say when the doctor might call?'

'She said he would try to come up this evening, but he might not manage until tomorrow morning, sir. He has other patients to attend to tonight.'

Charles nodded.

'Can I bring you some supper, sir?'

'Yes, Martha. Just put it on a tray. I'll eat here.'

'And the mistress, sir?'

'She's still sleeping. Best to leave her.'

'Very well, sir.'

Martha gifted her master a perfunctory bob and went down to the kitchen to warm the chops and potatoes that Mrs Drysdale had left on the kitchen bunker.

7

∼ Friday, 28 February 1817:
High Street, Edinburgh ∼

As soon as Robert stepped out of the prison, cold air scoured his throat. He folded his muffler tightly about his chest, buried his chin in its soft, dark-green wool.

He ought to hurry home for supper. Margaret would be wondering what had become of him. If he had not been in the Tolbooth, a full day of schooling would now be under his belt. He would have taught his pupils arithmetic and Bible study in the morning and, after lunch, history and grammar. His correspondence would have been completed, and by now he would have been in the main hall saying grace over the evening meal.

And yet, he dawdled all the way down towards St Mary's Wynd, the day's events jostling for position in his head. While he felt partially satisfied with the pattern of communication he had established with Jean, he was frustrated by the patience needed to enable her to open up to him. Lord Succoth wanted answers and Robert suspected the judge would have little patience for anything that he deemed peripheral to the case.

What he needed was a whisky. A dram would warm and relax him.

Robert didn't drink as a rule. There were no spirits in his home or in the school. At formal functions, he would take a glass to be amiable but, in general, he liked to monitor the face he presented to the world. Maggie often teased him for being too strait-laced and, while he envied her sense of fun and easy way with people, his attempts at following her lead always felt forced. He wasn't entirely sure why that was. Perhaps he was worried that excess alcohol might threaten his carefully constructed edifice of propriety.

No matter. He was decided. This evening called for a whisky.

Robert juked into an inn at the top of the Canongate. It was adequate, a place frequented by tradesmen and travellers. When he pushed open the timber door, there were no more than half a dozen people in the small room. A group of middle-aged men and a young, well-to-do couple. Kinniburgh tipped his hat to his fellow patrons and made for a quiet corner. A small, fair-haired girl approached him from an inner room, and he gave her his order.

After a few moments, the girl returned, took a cloth from her apron to wipe a glass and poured a measure of whisky from an earthenware decanter.

He sat in an inglenook nursing his glass. A narrow leaded window looked onto the street and Robert could see the distorted shapes of passers-by, their elongated shadows cast by a street lantern. He fished a small notebook from his greatcoat pocket and smoothed it flat beside him on the stone seat. He took a pencil from his jacket. Proper note-making being an impossibility in the midst of signed conversation, his interview with Jean had given him little opportunity to make any written observations, so he was keen to jot down anything that might be important before the details of the day faded from memory. Robert lifted the glass and drank a mouthful of the thin, harsh liquid. It both scorched and soothed on the way down.

Robert had been much struck by Jean's recollection of her childhood. Yesterday, on his way to the Tolbooth –

34

perhaps as a result of the contents of Succoth's letter – he had constructed a very fixed view of this female prisoner he was destined to meet. A picture had formed in his mind of someone very different to him, someone to be pitied or condemned. But, when Jean had talked of her childhood in Islay, particularly about her parents and siblings, he couldn't help but be carried back to his own beginnings.

He had been born in 1780, in the small Dunbartonshire town of Kirkintilloch. His father, Walter, was a flax dresser and worked in a steady but piecemeal fashion from their small cottage and yard. His mother, Catherine, had borne and raised five children, all of whom thrived, including Robert. As the children grew older, they were set to work at the flax, under the supervision of his father, with heckle combs, separating the fibres of the plant and gathering up the resulting material to be delivered to the many weavers in the area. It was a lean existence but not without its pleasures. Robert and his brothers hunted rabbits and grouse in the fields around the town and, on market days, accompanied their father while he met with other tradesmen. While Walter bartered and socialised in the local coffee houses and drinking dens, the boys would venture into the swarm of people buying and selling next to the cross.

Robert was an exceptionally clever child and his mother managed to inveigle him a place at a local school, under the tutelage of the minister, Mr Watt, where he was by far the poorest social specimen. Nevertheless, he was amazed to discover that he could pick up Latin and Greek and History and Bible Studies better than all of the other boys, despite his humble background. The minister was similarly astonished and continued to oversee Robert's education and advancement in the absence of any remuneration.

'Can I get you another, sir?'

The fair-haired girl stood in front of him.

'Yes,' Robert replied, 'thank you.'

She smiled and poured another whisky into his glass. One of the group of men beckoned her over and began settling their bill, albeit in a rather chaotic, tipsy manner. The girl smiled indulgently and patiently counted out and reckoned the dribs and drabs of coins proffered by various members of the party. Satisfied their debt had been honoured, the men donned their coats and hats, jostled and joked at the door and were duly absorbed into the dark of the evening.

Robert brought his attention back to the notebook and the events of this afternoon. Jean had signed clearly, beautifully at times. She used basic signs that were in common with Robert's own, as well as others that appeared to have been learnt in Glasgow. The language they shared had been helpful and, although signs that were foreign to them presented an initial barrier, it was easily got over. Obstacles remained, certainly, but the essence of a signed language was there, and that fact fascinated him.

It was the means of communication that mattered, thought Robert, not the detail. This was what he found liberating. This was what he wished to convey to those people who saw the deaf making signs and judged their language inferior.

He had fallen into the teaching of the deaf, it was not a career that he had sought out, but the practical application of the methods he had learnt in London and Paris made him question the orthodoxies of the instruction of the deaf and dumb every day.

Now, here was a woman who faced the noose for that most unnatural of crimes, murder of her own child. A deaf woman with a story to tell. A story, it would seem, that only Robert Kinniburgh had any chance of interpreting.

The extrication of this tale and his ability to relay it in a way that a court could understand and make judgement upon must be his focus. Maybe it was the second whisky on an ill-prepared stomach, but Robert had a feeling there was more to Jean Campbell than the kind of tale of woe written up as a broadside ballad and sold for a penny by a street-corner chapman.

8

It was almost pitch black in the cell. A shaft of moonlight squeezed through the small opening in the wall, casting its beam upon the rough woollen blanket. Jean watched its shape alter as she shifted her feet, rubbing them to keep warm. Cold air seeped into the prison and turned liquid on the wall. The bed, jammed into a far corner, was a poor refuge, but it was all that was available to her. She tried to make the best of it by keeping her clothes on, and adding her shawl and an extra knitted coverlet that Mr Sibbald had given her to the scant bedclothes.

Her mind, as ever, was on Sandy. She had no idea where he was, and nights were when it was hardest to bear. Jean knew it was possible that her son was still with Jim Donnelly. She occasionally imagined him warm and sheltered in her aunt and uncle's home in the Calton. But this was a forlorn hope. If he was in the care of someone who knew her, surely she would have had word by now? He had been in the police office at Glasgow, Jean remembered. Or had she dreamt that? Sandy's pale-blue eyes looking at her in terror. She must have looked a fright, right enough, face bloodied and clothes torn. She couldn't quite make sense of what had happened after the bridge.

This man, Robert, had given his promise to help her. He had the power to ask questions and demand answers, but she would need to give him something in return. All she had to barter were her sins.

Jean's breasts ached under her loosened stays. A surfeit of milk for a baby that could no longer suckle. It hurt to touch. Years ago, when she had struggled, at first, to feed Sandy, her aunt had placed cabbage leaves next to her skin to draw out the milk and ease the pain. There was no one here to bring her any relief. Only a succession of men who wouldn't have known what she was asking, even if she could make the request understood.

She would ask Robert about Sandy, though. She had to make sure he was safe. Another loss would be too hard to bear.

9

~ *Saturday 1 March 1817:*
Saltmarket, Glasgow ~

Jim Donnelly woke up sober. In fact, despite a concerted attempt the night before, he had gone to bed sober as well. More or less. He had slept in his shirt and grey woollen socks. The room was bitterly cold outside of the warm bedding, so he pulled on his trousers and wrapped himself in one of the blankets. He lit a fire in the grate and heated some water to make a cup of tea. The end of a small loaf of bread lay uncovered on the settle. It was hard, but Jim chewed on it anyway.

He let the door bang behind him and went down a flight of steps outside the building to the courtyard below. It was just as cold outside the room and the smell of shite in the open sewer not as bad as it was during the warmer summer months. He walked out of Taylor's Close on to Goosedub's Lane and turned into the Briggait, where limpid sunlight bathed his face. Then he walked towards the Old Bridge, in the expectation that the boatman would be resuming his search.

The Humane Society had a cottage on Glasgow Green, on the north shore of the Clyde, where Mr Duncan, the boatman, maintained boats and equipment for the prevention of waterway accidents and the rescue of persons in distress. Almost a week after the event, the boatman was still trawling for evidence on the orders of the sergeant of the Bridge-end Police Office.

When the cry had gone up last Monday evening and crowds had gathered to watch the spectacle, Jean was apprehended and taken into the custody of the sergeant. The next morning, Mr Duncan, assisted by a medical student from the university, had ventured onto the river. Although they were in daylight, it was misty, dark and the blackened water of the Clyde clasped its treasures tightly. Even an experienced boatman like Mr Duncan struggled in the fog; it not only made visibility difficult, but deadened sound and played strange tricks so that it became impossible to tell which direction noises were coming from. The pair had continued looking well into the night, making trips back to the boathouse to replenish their lanterns and warm themselves up by Mr Duncan's fire. Eventually, they had to admit defeat but, after a few hours' sleep and a warm breakfast courtesy of the boatman's wife, they had started again on the Wednesday morning. When nothing was found, the baby was relegated to the list of missing and incorporated into the boatman's daily round.

~

Jim had spent much of the previous day in an ale house on the Saltmarket. Rarely the most convivial customer, Big Nell, the landlady, and a few of the other patrons felt enough pity or curiosity to stand him the odd small beer.

Donnelly was a fellow who said little as a rule. When drunk, however, he said a lot, much of it easy to take offence at, and he was often seen brawling as a result. Today, despite the alcohol, he was subdued. Not surprising really, since his bidie-in had been carted off to Edinburgh and the mystery baby was still missing, presumed dead.

Jim had been in this state for days. God only knew how he was funding his extended pub crawl. A man like him needed regular work to pay for his board and lodging and Jim had not been seen for hire all this time. He was a labourer and, since arriving in the city ten years ago, was accustomed to take any work going. Whether it was on the canal or down at the docks, there was always something needing tearing down or putting up. Glasgow and its environs were in a constant state of flux as they tried to cope with the movement of people and goods in and out of the city.

He pushed his tumbler forward and Big Nell ambled over to him.

'Another one, James?' Nell asked him, raising her eyebrows to question, and yet abdicate responsibility for, the wisdom of him having another.

Jim nodded.

'Whisky, Nell,' slurred the Irishman.

Nell nodded her head and poured a dram into his glass. She set the whisky down on the bar and gathered up her customer's proffered payment.

'Any news of Jean?' she asked.

Jim shook his head. 'I've heard nothing since they took her through-by.'

'And where did you hear about that?'

Jim jerked his head in the direction of the river. 'From the sergeant at the Bridge-end.'

Nell leant across the bar. 'Was that the same day they arrested her?'

'No. She was in the Bridge-end jail from the Monday till the Wednesday. Not that I saw her, Nell. Bastards wouldn't let me over the door.'

Jim took a gulp of the whisky and closed his eyes.

'First I knew that anything had happened was when I got back from work on the Monday night. I came over from the Gorbals side of the river and I saw a wee crowd outside the jail, but I never paid any attention. See when I got home now, I knew something was wrong. The wee man was breaking his heart and Jean wasn't there.'

Nell took a breath and shook her head.

'That's no like Jean, eh? She cares for that wean good as anybody.'

Jim considered this for a moment.

'Aye, fair enough, but she'd already left the boy for weeks.'

'Where's wee Sandy now?' Nell asked.

Jim shrugged.

'Had to take him to the parish. How am I going to look after him?'

Nell murmured an assent but averted her eyes. A land-lady knew better than to pass comment on the domestic arrangements of her patrons.

Her customer sat looking at his empty whisky glass, but he didn't ask for another.

~

Now, Jim sat on a pillar on the dry dock just under the Old Bridge. The boatman had not arrived yet. Jim knew he would enter the water a few yards further east and row under the low wooden bridge, casting his gaze from side to side as he approached the place where Jim sat. Jim would see him by and by. The surface of the water was grey, a weak sun coaxing occasional glints of silver. The city was waking up and a few men were unloading crates from a small craft. They paid him no attention.

Jim felt for the coins in his pocket and thought about Jean and the wee fella. She was far away from him now. If they hanged her, he'd never see her again. It was likely that Sandy was at the parish, but Jim hadn't taken him there, despite what he'd said to Nell. The police had come around, found the lad alone and taken him away for questioning. Why would they return him? Jim wasn't his father, just like he wasn't Jean's husband. He had simply wandered into their lives fully expecting to wander back out again. Now that the baby was gone, he was little more than a spectator.

10

~ Monday, 24 February 1817:
Briggait, Glasgow ~

The Glasgow police had been at a loss as to how to deal with this silent woman. The crowd that gathered on the police office steps immediately following the incident needed to be dispersed so that any crime could be established, investigated properly and a search got underway. As the sergeant remonstrated with the mob, one of their number piped up.

'No point asking that yin anything!'

This proved to be the case. Despite the best efforts of the police and some assistance from a couple of worthies from the Trades Hall, no one was found who could induce the woman to tell them what had occurred on the bridge. A sensible fellow from Barclay's Rope and Soapworks, who was a deaf man himself and who had a bit of speech, spoke to Jean patiently and at length but she simply shrank into herself.

'Does she understand the signs you're making?' the sergeant asked, impatient for progress.

'I can't tell, sir,' the Barclay's man replied. 'I'm sorry.'

The man's voice and accent sounded strange to the sergeant's ears. Not Glaswegian, exactly, and the pitch of it lurched in an unexpected manner. The sergeant thanked him for his time and sent him back to the works with a note for his employer.

On the Tuesday, his silent prisoner appeared in court

and the sergeant was forced to admit defeat. Thereafter, a decision was made to send her to Edinburgh, where a young man called Kinniburgh was reported to be achieving great things in the education of deaf and dumb children.

11

～ Sunday, 2 January 1814:
Calton, Glasgow ～

During the first week of every month, the Society for the Deaf and Dumb held a church service and social. The New Year's Day event was always well attended, with people wishing to prolong the convivial atmosphere that came with ringing in the bells of a fresh year.

It was Jean's Aunt Nancy that had first heard of the place. Nancy that mentioned it to her own minister, who nodded and said he knew something of the man in charge. An older chap by the name of Buchanan and his wife, who had a deaf son of their own, had started the Society as a means of preaching to those who could not hear sermons. Why should a quirk of fate keep those afflicted by deafness from the word of God? Apparently, some of the merchants and businessmen had gifted a little money to keep the enterprise afloat and were in the process of forming a committee they hoped might help it flourish. Nancy's minister thought it a good idea for her to take her niece along.

Aunt Nancy was a practical woman. It wasn't Jean's mortal soul that she was primarily concerned with but how her niece and young Sandy might fare in the long term. Jean would need to find some means of making a living if she wanted to keep hold of the wee soul and the best way to do that was to get to know folk. Her uncle and aunt would help out, but the two rooms and kitchen that Bill and Nancy rented in James Street Lane were already crowded and couldn't sustain another family indefinitely. This was the way it was for now, though. They had promised Bill's sister to look after her daughter until she was on her feet again.

Nancy was fond of her niece and had known her since infancy. They rubbed along just fine. Jean helped with the housework and was good at keeping the smaller children occupied while Nancy got on with cooking and washing. Nancy knew some of the signs that Jean used; was surprised at how many of them she remembered from before she and Bill had left Islay. In the main, however, she relied on lip-speaking to communicate and, when all else failed, Nancy would draw a picture with anything that was to hand. Sometimes in the flour as she made pastry or on the condensation on the kitchen window. She wasn't much of a draughtswoman and the weans laughed at her efforts, but she and Jean could usually make sense of the world together.

~

The church lay back from the street between two tall houses. It was a squat wooden building with scrolled writing carved into a lintel above a doorway. Lights burned, yellow in the gloom, from two square leaded windows either side of the entrance. Aunt Nancy stopped and reached out her hand to tuck a stray strand of hair back under Jean's shawl. She looked her niece straight in the eye and smiled.

Nancy fanned out the fingers of her right hand, twirled them briefly, before grasping them back into a fist.

Beautiful. Ready?

Are you not coming with me?

Aunt Nancy shook her head and lifted two fingers to her ear. *I'm not deaf, hen. I don't think they'll have me.*

She patted Jean's arm and pointed. *Away you inside. It'll be grand. I'll come back for you at nine.*

Nancy thrust four fingers out horizontally to signal the time. Then wagged her finger.

Don't you be leaving me waiting outside in this cold, mind.

Nancy squeezed her elbows in to her sides to indicate a shiver.

The women embraced and Jean turned towards the doorway. She squared her shoulders and walked inside.

It was a small church, simply furnished. A narrow central aisle with perhaps a dozen pews on either side; an open area at the front, where a large Bible lay on a pulpit. Beside it, a small man in black dress and clerical collar, strands of sandy hair swept over a bald pate, was deep in conversation with a group of parishioners. No more than thirty people peppered the wooden pews. A middle-aged lady, standing near the minister, noticed Jean and walked purposefully towards her. She tapped Jean's elbow.

Hello. You're very welcome. Would you like to sit down? The service is about to start.

Jean nodded, and the lady ushered her into a pew. Two other women were already there, and they smiled and shuffled along to make space. Jean nodded a thank you and slipped into her place. A small ledge protruded from the back of the row in front of her and she tapped the tips of her fingers on it for a moment, then pulled her arms down to her sides, resting her palms on the cool, smooth surface of the pale wood.

A length of heavy embroidery hung on the far wall. On it, a bearded saint in plain brown robes, knotted with rope, stood over a young boy. The saint held a book in his hand and the boy gazed up at him. It was an ordinary scene but for the shards of light that emanated from the haloed man's feet and hands and from an unlikely gash in his chest.

Jean's eyes were drawn to the luminous thread that shone, miraculous, in the candlelight.

There was a short flurry of activity as people settled down in their seats and the minister waved his hands in the air to get everyone's attention. He gestured a welcome and made a sign for them to pray. Jean clasped her hands together in her lap and made to bow her head. To her surprise, the congregation looked straight ahead with their eyes wide open. Jean followed suit.

The minister began to pray.

Thank you, Lord, for your love and kindness. For keeping us safe this long winter. For all your blessings of nature and industry. We ask you, Lord, to help us, your children, in all we do. To bless us with food and shelter in this new year and all the years to come.

The prayers were full of thanks and the minister duly tapped, tapped, tapped his pale clergyman's fingers on his chin and offered up his palms to the Almighty.

Jean was delighted to discover that she understood the gist of what he was saying. She had always been taught to bow her head when others did and would be nudged by her parents when it was time to look up again. In this church, nothing was withheld from her, and she could follow a prayer for the first time. The signs were not completely familiar to her, but in some cases they were very close to the hand gestures she used with her family and friends. Even the signs she didn't recognise were often easy to guess at. Growing up, she had spent enough time at church to pick up the thread of common prayers and hymns. She had followed the lip patterns of the minister and the congregation and copied her parents and brothers as they learnt their Bible stories.

Reverend Buchanan gestured to the congregation to rise and everyone got to their feet. He pointed heavenward and made the sign for *shepherd* by shaping the outline of a crook and standing to attention. The assembly began to sign the hymn, and Jean joined in.

The Lord is my shepherd, I'll not want. He makes me down to lie, in pastures green.

She remembered the rhythm and a few of the words, at least in the first couple of verses. She watched as the minister produced handshapes for the words she didn't know, determined to remember them for next time.

The Reverend Buchanan next beckoned to a man sitting in the front of the congregation and he stood up and took his place next to the minister. The man was plainly dressed and had a shock of thick grey hair that curled up where it touched his shirt collar. He looked like a weaver or a joiner, constrained in a rarely worn jacket that had become too tight for him. The minister introduced him as George and the man began to sign a story.

Jesus travelled to Galilee and passed a land where there were ten cities. Here, some people brought him a man who could neither hear nor speak and they begged Jesus to touch him. Instead, Jesus put his fingers into the deaf man's ears and then spat on his own finger and laid it on the deaf man's tongue.

The deaf people in the church concentrated hard as George signed the story. The facial expressions he adopted while describing the deaf character in the story made his audience laugh out loud, and the minister, rather than issuing a reprimand, chuckled along with them. George made the deaf man seem like an ordinary fellow such as you might meet whistling on his way to work in the morning or staggering out of a nearby inn having spent too much of his wages on drink. George's Jesus was a kindly passer-by, stopping to help his neighbour, despite the urgency of his own journey.

51

Jean watched George and her fellow churchgoers, fascinated by their involvement in this entertaining story and struck by how different this service was to any other she had known. For once, she didn't need to copy her neighbour's reactions or to sit still, worried that she would embarrass herself or those she was with. The two women sitting next to her were laughing and nodding along, making signs that George then repeated. Jean wondered if this was a story that they all knew.

The man was healed, he could hear and began to talk. It seemed impossible. The people were amazed. Jesus asked them not to say anything about what he had done but the crowd could not stop talking about it. It was a miracle that should be shared across the land.

Here George made a play of producing a declaration that he rounded up into a scroll and unfurled in the manner of a town crier. He thrust out his chest and puffed up his cheeks, transforming himself into a self-important city servant. Then, just as quickly, he seemed to deflate and become one member of the crowd after another, whispering and chattering until he painted the air thick with gossip.

When he was simply George again, the minister squeezed his shoulders. Everyone was clapping and signing to George and to each other.

He's a caution, so he is!

Well done, well done.

A good story well told.

The minister stood still, waiting for them to bring their attention back to the front of the church.

Jesus had just performed a miracle. Why did he not want the people to talk about it?

Jean didn't know. It was strange. Stranger still for a minister to ask his congregation a question that he appeared to want them to answer.

The Reverend Buchanan looked out at his congregation. *Why did Jesus perform miracles?*

~

After a closing prayer, the service came to an end and the Reverend Buchanan's wife made an announcement. They were all very welcome to stay for something to eat and drink. She opened the door to a back room, where tables and chairs were covered with linen cloths and set with embroidered napkins. Mrs Buchanan and some of the ladies shuttled back and forth from a small kitchen area, laying out plates of cakes and sandwiches and serving hot tea to the assembly.

Jean hung back. A tall woman wearing a mustard-coloured bonnet approached her and guided her to a table where two women and a man were happily installed, sharing out shortbread and scones.

The lady in the mustard hat caught their attention and asked, *Will you look after this new girl?*

The man stood up to let Jean take her seat and signed to her. *You're deaf, yes? You know sign?*

Jean nodded but gestured to explain she didn't understand everything.

The man laughed and patted her hand. *Don't you worry, we'll show you what's what.*

12

Jean blew on her hands. A meagre fire guttered in the stale air, and any warmth that gathered soon evaporated, escaping from the thin window and a huge gap between the old wood of the door and the worn flagstones beneath it.

She and Robert sat in the cell. He on a wooden chair, resting his arm on the table, and she perched at the fireplace.

I began to know the deaf of the city. All my life, I had relied on my family to look after me. When I met other people who were like me, I felt like I belonged. Her eyes brimmed with tears at the memory.

Robert shook his head, sadly. *It is a hard thing to be forced to communicate in someone else's language.* Robert moved his hands back and forth with bent thumbs and index fingers, to signify a conversation.

Yes, to always be the one who is lacking. Jean brought the fingers of both hands together, pulled them apart from each other and let them fall.

But, that first time at the church. They made you feel welcome, didn't they?

She nodded, *They did. It was a surprise, how much of their signing I understood.*

How did you understand it, asked Robert *when you had only made up your own signs within your small family?*

It's hard to explain. Jean considered for a moment. *The people at the church were kind and patient. I didn't know each sign, but the way they spoke made sense. It was as if the world had always been in sign language. I just hadn't learnt it.*

Jean shivered.

Are you cold? Robert asked.

A little.

Robert walked across the cell and lifted a blanket from a basket in the corner. It was old, and the pattern faded to almost nothing, but it smelt clean. He handed it to Jean, and she laid it across her lap, tucking the ends under her skirt.

I think deaf language is very different. It is something you can see.

Do you mean like a picture? asked Robert.

Jean thought for a moment. *Yes, but more than a picture. It is full of movement, like a dance or an entertainment. Where I live, there are stalls on fair days at Glasgow Green. Men tell a story to the crowd. They tell stories about kings and soldiers and criminals.*

Robert had also seen these tellers of tales. At fair days in the Grassmarket and on the Meadows in Edinburgh. Balladeers recited stories full of grisly violence and salacious detail. The crowds, very few of whom could write their own name never mind read a newspaper or a book, flocked to hear about men who cut up their wives and knife-wielding gangs that rampaged through the cities. Robert could not comprehend why these cowed and exploited people, most of whom lived hand to mouth in the midst of the factories and workshops and slums, would wish to immerse themselves in more suffering and violence than they knew already.

These stories are outrageous, he said. *They show the people everything that is wicked in this life.*

Jean looked at him in surprise. *But people pay to watch them.*

They do, he agreed. *People might be better off concentrating on higher things.*

Jean shrugged. *Higher things are written down. Higher things are written in books, not acted out in the streets. It is not real. When I met the deaf in Glasgow, they were able to show me the stories of life, not just tell them.*

She shook her index and middle finger downwards. *Not just repeat the same thing again and again.*

Robert thought about what she had said.

At the school where I am the master, many deaf children are delighted to meet their fellows. They share a common sensibility, one which, perhaps, they did not have at home with their families.

Don't they miss their families? Jean asked.

Yes, especially at the beginning, but when they settle in, they often remark on how easy they find communication with the other pupils. It seems to relieve an anxiety that is always present when they are with people who can hear. Even with those who love and care for them.

That is how I felt. I had been missing something. I didn't know what it was until I found it.

Robert brought his two index fingers together. *Meeting people who are the same as you is a great liberation from the cares of the world.*

Yes, I felt a connection and saw that I was only different from hearing people, not worse than them.

Robert paused and steadied himself. *I need to ask you about what happened to your baby.*

I know. Jean drew a hand from under her shawl and patted her breast, as if she were trying to damp down some emotion that threatened to overcome her.

Robert ducked his head and met her gaze.

It is you who I am here to speak for. No one else.

She did not respond.

You told me that nobody would believe you. I will believe you and explain your story to the court.

She shifted slightly in her seat.

But if I have committed a crime?

Then I will try to tell the court the truth of it. If it was an accident, they may look kindly upon you.

Jean shook her head. *It was no accident.*

Then tell me what it was. I cannot advise your lawyers how best to represent you, if I do not know what you have done and why you have done it.

I don't know how to, Jean said, moving her outstretched palms towards him in a circling motion to represent the unfolding of a story.

Start at the beginning, Robert told her.

She pulled herself upright and pursed her lips.

As I told you before, I came to Glasgow to live with my aunt and uncle when I had my son. I named him Sandy. At this, Jean made a sign by holding up her right hand and rubbing her thumb over her fingertips.

Like sand? Robert smiled.

Yes. That was his sign name. They told me I had named my boy after my father, but I didn't understand that at first. My father had the name Alec, but he was always just my father to me. She stretched out the index and middle fingers of both hands and tapped them together. *But his name comes from the same place as Sandy. I didn't mean to do it, but it seemed like a good omen. Do you have a sign name?*

I remember that, yesterday, you referred to me as the clean-shaven one. Robert mimicked the motion Jean had made by stroking his cheek twice.

She laughed at this. *I remember. But that is also the sign for a woman. And, where I come from, it also means a molly. It is not polite.*

Robert blushed. He knew what a molly was, but it was

not a word or a subject that he was in the habit of discussing, especially with a woman. Jean's blithe reference to men who went with men was not something he was used to.

Jean seemed to sense his embarrassment. *So, tell me your Sunday sign name.*

Robert lip-spoke his first name and made the sign for a teacher by moving his curled index fingers outwards from his mouth. Usually, the fingers were not curled but straight. However, this shape mimicked the finger-spelling for the letter R, combining both his Christian name and his occupation.

And you? he asked.

Jean pinched her thumb and forefinger together, fanned out the rest of her fingers. She drew a circle in the air between them two or three times.

Robert smiled. *The Island One.*

The island is in the past. Jean gestured with her hand, pushed her flat palm over her shoulder to indicate that this period in her life was now history. And yet, her hand wavered, as if she was reluctant to let it go.

Would you go back?

If they'd have me. I'm not sure I still belong there.

The cell door opened and Sibbald appeared, carrying a battered tin tray of victuals. He acknowledged Robert and Jean and set his cargo on the table.

'I've brung you bread and cheese, sir. And small beer to revive you,' said the keeper.

'Thank you, Mr Sibbald, it's much appreciated,' said Robert.

'Aye, well, Mr Kinniburgh, sir, I can't claim to have prepared it myself. Up until a few months ago, we had a woman who came in to cook and prepare meals for the prisoners, but since we've been headed for the knacker's yard, it's only me that the burghers pay to be of use.'

58

'Well, it's good of you to go to the trouble.' Robert looked at the contents of the tray. A decent-looking portion of fresh loaf accompanied by a rather sweaty chunk of Cheddar and a generous jug of small beer would suffice and see them through the afternoon.

Sibbald had started his tale, and so continued.

'I cannae cook to save my life, sir, so it's just as well they give me an allowance to provide what's needed. I got this from the inn that belongs to Mrs Candlish. You might know it, sir, it's just across the way.'

'I'm not sure I do, Mr Sibbald. I'm not often in the High Street.'

'Aye, you're probably best biding down the Canongate, Mr Kinniburgh. The High Street can be a rough place at times. Although, I have to say, Mrs Candlish runs a gey respectable establishment. Fine woman she is and all.'

'It looks a fine repast. Please thank Mrs Candlish on my behalf. Can I give you anything for your trouble?'

Sibbald held up his hand to wave away the suggestion, 'Not at all, sir. As I said, I have an allowance to cover such things. We are above board, in this respect, you and I.'

Robert lifted the knife and began to carve slices from the loaf.

'What will happen to you, Mr Sibbald, when the Tolbooth closes?' asked Robert. 'Will you be given work at the new prison?'

'No, sir. I'm getting too old for that carry-on. Me and the wife have our eye on a housekeeping position in Cramond. Fresh air and peace and quiet in our old age. I've had enough of villains, sir' – he looked shamefaced and turned to Jean for a second – 'present company excepted, of course.'

Jean glanced at him and Robert caught her gaze, as if to say, don't worry, there is nothing of import being said.

Still, he noticed that she kept watching them, trying perhaps to lip-read some of their conversation, interpreting more by their body language.

Robert cut the cheese into chunks, poured two tumblers from the jug and passed one to Jean. He placed the large plate between them and gestured to her to eat.

'It sounds a fine plan, Mr Sibbald. Getting out of the old town. Progress seems to be abandoning us in its wake.'

Robert, still chewing on a mouthful of his lunch, turned to Jean and signed, *They are building a new prison to the north-west of the city, Mr Sibbald's job will disappear.*

I am sorry for that.

No need, Mr Sibbald and his wife are escaping to a beautiful place just outside Edinburgh. A village of industry and wealth. I am sure they will do well there.

Sibbald shifted awkwardly on his feet throughout this exchange.

'Would you like to sit down, Mr Sibbald?' asked Robert.

'No, sir, I'll be off and leave you to it. I'll bring you some coffee in a while.'

'Thank you,' acknowledged Robert.

When Sibbald was gone, Jean took a gulp of her beer and smiled conspiratorially. *Do you think Mr Sibbald has a sign name?*

Robert was confused. *He doesn't know the deaf, how could he?*

But if he did. I know what it might be.

What?

Jean pushed out her cheeks and twirled an imaginary set of keys around a finger.

Robert laughed despite himself.

Jean covered her mouth.

I'm sorry. I should not make fun of him. He is a good

man. *Kind. A woman alone in this place could be taken advantage of.*

Robert looked at her. *We are all trying to help you, Jean. Will you continue with your story?*

She inhaled deeply, as if steeling herself, worried that once she started to speak, she might not be able to stop.

For a few years, me and Sandy got on well. Money was always scarce. I worked at the mill. It was hard work.

Jean thrust her thumb against the palm of her outstretched left hand to indicate the extent of her labours.

If you weren't there on time, the gates were closed, and you'd get no money. But I got used to it and the other women were friendly.

They were happy to take a deaf woman on? Robert asked.

In a cotton mill, the noise can be fierce, she explained. *Being deaf didn't make much difference.*

You made friends at the deaf church? Robert asked.

Yes, said Jean, *I went to the church two or three times a week. The service on a Sunday and there were meetings in the evenings where you could practise making signs.*

You didn't learn the alphabet or how to make sounds?

Jean shook her head. *Some of the children did. The minister taught them. The adults were more interested in signing with each other.*

But being able to speak and to know how to spell, would that not make it easier for you all to get on in the world?

Jean thought about this for a moment. *When you try to speak, people laugh at you.*

Robert understood. *In my school, we teach in English and try to help the pupils read lips and make speech. I let them sign amongst themselves outside of the classroom. Some teachers disagree and punish those who sign.*

Jean looked shocked. *That's not fair.* She adopted a scowling expression and pointed at her neck, twisting her finger to indicate the cruelty of this course of action. *When I went to the meetings in the church, I was able to understand and be understood. It felt like a huge burden had been taken from me.*

You were happy, then? asked Robert.

Jean nodded earnestly.

What changed? he asked. *Why were you living apart from your aunt and uncle when the police arrested you?*

I met a man.

Can you tell me this man's name?

Jean thought for a second, then mouthed the name Jim.

You were living with Jim. Is he your husband? Robert asked.

Jean blushed. *He has given me a ring.*

Robert glanced at her left hand. There was no ring there.

Have you been married in a church?

No. He is Catholic and I am Protestant so there is no one to marry us.

Robert tried to conceal his distaste. She seemed such a decent woman despite her poor clothes and lack of education. The word 'hoor' kept returning to him. Succoth had called her that and only yesterday Jean herself had said that someone might use it to refer to her. She was living in sin with this man, she was not stupid and must realise that this was wrong, and yet she presented the arrangement as perfectly normal. He wondered if this was all bluff on her part, the mention of a ring a curious defence against immorality.

Jean carried on. *My aunt and uncle weren't happy, that I'd taken up with an Irishman. It made a great rift between us. I went to live with Jim in the Saltmarket.*

Jean paused, thinking for a moment, and then made a handshape for the street name. Her fingers mimicked a sprinkling motion and then both hands affected a kind of half-opened fist that she moved back and forth, suggesting trading and movement.

What about your wee boy? Robert asked.

I left him with my aunt and kept going to my work. I called round to see him when my uncle wasn't there. My Uncle Bill was angry, he said I had disgraced the family. She shrugged. *I'd disgraced my father and now my uncle.* Jean's expression was one of inevitability and regret. *Aunt Nancy said I should give Jim up. But I couldn't. One day, my uncle came home early and found me there. He told me not to come again. I took Sandy and we both stayed with Jim from then on.*

Did the baby belong to Jim?

Jean nodded. *What is it they say, lightning can't strike twice? Well, it turned out that it could.*

She rolled her eyes, and Robert didn't know where to put himself. It was such a shameful thing. Not only to be unmarried in the eyes of God but to bring a bastard into the world. Jean poured them both another tumbler of beer from the jug and took another slice of bread and cheese. Robert did likewise, and they ate in silence for a few minutes. Jean looked vacantly into the middle distance, but she seemed to be turning over the events of the previous year in her head.

Robert wondered at what she had told him so far. An unwanted pregnancy and a possible solution that ended so badly that she hardly knew how to frame it in her own head, never mind explain it to a man who was considered so much better than her.

She finished eating and began to sign again. *If I had known how difficult my life would become, I might not have been so headstrong.* She bunched her fists together and jolted them to demonstrate her wilfulness in throwing in her lot with Jim.

63

Why was it so difficult?

I had no one to protect me. I lost my job because I had nowhere to put Sandy. People would not speak to me as long as I was with Jim.

Why did you stay with him, then?

Because I wanted him, she stated, boldly. *I couldn't imagine a life where I wasn't able to lie in bed with him.*

Robert looked away. He felt such an acute sense of humiliation, and yet he was not the one who had said the shameful thing.

13

∼ Saturday, 21 September 1816:
Taylor's Close, Glasgow ∼

Jim Donnelly and Jean Campbell lay tangled in sheets
that were so patched and threadbare, little of the original
material remained. An ill-fitting sash and case window
had been raised. Dust motes drifted up from the yard
below and tumbled around in shafts of yellow sunlight.
Jean could faintly discern a repetitive clang from the
blacksmith's workshop at the entrance to the close. Jim
could hear women gossiping and laughing while they
hauled water from the communal well to begin the day's
washing.

Jean pulled herself up into a sitting position and clambered over Jim. She took the cracked chamber pot from
underneath the bed and squatted over it to urinate. As the
months had worn on, the pressure of the baby on her
bladder had increased and she seemed to need to piss every
few minutes, even though she produced barely a trickle. It
had been about five months since she had stopped bleeding
and her belly was rounded now. Jean had sewn extra panels
into her skirt to make life more comfortable but to lie in
bed naked all the warm morning was a rare kind of liberation. She would have to get dressed in order to empty
the pot and collect some water before long, but she climbed
back into bed for the present.

Jim reached over and rubbed his hand across her taut
belly. Jean turned towards him, thinking he wanted to fuck

again, but he pointed at his wilted cock and shook his head ruefully.

He's on strike, he mouthed at her. *You've worn him out.*

His laughter at this turn of events shook through her.

That was him all over, Jean thought. Joking, drinking, carrying on. Working a few days to pay for the next round of revelry. It was all very well for a time, but how could she look after herself and Sandy and a new baby on laughter?

Jean reached down and clutched at his arm. The black hairs on his forearm distracted her from her anxiety momentarily but she pushed back desire and made an effort to concentrate on practicalities.

She shook her head and used her right hand to signify laughter. *It's not funny.*

Jim put his arm around her shoulder. *You have to laugh, sure.*

He watched as she shook her head again. He couldn't tell if she was angry because he had misconstrued her meaning or if she was exercised about something else entirely. They probably understood around half of what each other were trying to say. A bit of lip-reading and a smattering of signs was an efficient enough method of communication for the practicalities of life. Feelings, hopes and expectations were another matter entirely.

It'll be alright, Jean. He leant over and kissed her, their dry lips sticking together. Instinctively, Jean lifted her pelvis to rub against his hand and felt annoyed with herself. Why was fucking so easy? Why was it such a sin? People had either to be good or bad and she no longer knew what category she fitted into.

She pushed herself back up into a sitting position.

What are we to do for money? She slapped the fingers of her right hand onto her left palm.

He shrugged. *Can you not go back to your family? They took you in before.*

No, she pursed her lips, *this is different. They'll have nothing to do with papists.* She made the sign of a cross at her forehead. Although this was also the sign for Catholic, her expression suggested the wholly negative way in which Irish immigrants like Jim were viewed by the largely Protestant populace.

He glared at her.

They lay for a while, barely moving. Eventually, Jim lifted a pipe and a pouch of tobacco from the stool beside the bed and packed it down. He got up and lit it at the fire, pulling hard until it took.

She watched him, then she cast her palm in front of her face. *I'm sorry.*

It's alright. You're just speaking the truth.

I don't think that way. Do you know that?

He nodded. *I know.*

Jim had another puff of his pipe and passed it to Jean, who took a couple of draws and handed it back to him.

He drove both of his palms straight in front of him. *I'll be back on the canals next week. I'm trying, hen. I can only earn when there's work.*

She nodded an acknowledgment.

It's not enough, though. Not enough to feed you, me, Sandy and this wean when it comes. I don't know how we'll manage.

Jim put his arm around her. *The rent's paid till I get back. I can leave you a wee bit of money. Maybe you could get a few shifts at the mill?*

She pushed him away, furious. *Are you daft? Who'll look after Sandy while I'm working?*

Stillness enveloped them once more. All former passion turned sour. Reality had seeped into their bones.

After a few moments, Jean turned to him.

There's a hearing man comes to the Deaf Church sometimes. He has a yard at the docks in Partick. She made a sign for a boat or a ship and tweaked her nose upwards to signify his wealth and status. *Him and his wife live in a big house off the Dumbarton Road. She keeps losing her babies.*

14

∼ Saturday, 1 March 1817:
The Tolbooth Prison, Edinburgh ∼

Jean straightened and began. *Jim and me. We couldn't afford to have the baby. We could barely manage to feed ourselves on what he was earning. I couldn't get any work once my pregnancy became noticeable. At the Deaf Church, the man approached me with a solution.*

Who was the man?

I cannot say. I have no spelling. His sign name was like a boat on the river. Jean brought the fingertips of both her hands together and moved them forward. *He lived to the west of the city.*

Did he work at the docks?

No, I don't think so. He had a large house and a carriage. He went to work near the river. I think he built ships or moved goods.

A wealthy man?

Yes. A man of business. He was one of the people who gave money to the church.

What solution did he propose?

That he and his wife would take my baby. Jean brought her hands together in a cradling motion at her breast. *They could have none of their own.*

Robert was confused. Did she mean that the couple meant to take the baby from her? Was this something that Jean had done willingly? He splayed the fingers of his right hand, wrapped them around his left fist and pulled it into him. *They would adopt it?*

Jean shrugged. It was plain she didn't understand what the sign meant.

Robert tried to break the action down for her, present it as a story. *You were to have the child and then hand it over to them. Were you happy about that?*

She rolled her eyes in disdain at the suggestion. *Of course not, but this man seemed so sad about not having any children and he and his wife could give the baby a good start in life. I wasn't sure I would manage to feed it or keep it alive for any length of time. The state we were living in. I was only able to look after Sandy because my aunt and uncle had helped me. There was no chance of that anymore.*

And Jim Donnelly, Robert asked, *did he support this plan?*

Not at first. He was very angry when I first came to him with it. He wanted to provide for us, but he knew he couldn't. Jim has a good heart, but he drinks and fights too much and I knew I couldn't rely on him. I would rather give up my child than condemn it to a life on the streets. Jim made a fuss, but it was soon over.

Did this man and his wife suggest they pay you for the baby?

Jean's face flushed, but she gathered herself and explained.

We made an agreement. He offered me bed and board in my confinement. He said he would pay me one pound when the baby was born and, if I stayed on to nurse it for a few months after the birth, he would pay me a weekly wage. Then, as soon as the baby was thriving and had been weaned, he would give me another one pound upon leaving.

I see, Robert said. *That is a substantial sum of money.*

She looked at him defiantly. *I felt my baby was worth a substantial sum of money.*

Robert sat quietly for a few minutes, mulling this contract

70

over. He was considering not only the costs involved in this transaction, but the very nature of the bargain itself. To barter a child seemed unthinkable, but then he had never lived in the depths of poverty that Jean had known since she had thrown in her lot with Donnelly. A sum of that kind, if used wisely, would offer an escape for her and her son. He wondered if that was what she had in mind when she had entered into this transaction, or if Donnelly himself had cajoled her for his own ends, his eye on the main chance.

You accepted the offer? he asked.

Jean nodded.

It was near the end of my pregnancy. I could feel the baby lying lower in my belly and become still. I knew the birth was close. I walked to the house with Jim.

Where was this house?

We followed the river and walked up a hill in the west. Jean made a sign that Robert didn't recognise; she pinched her thumb and forefinger together and drew them towards her temple, flicking them outwards at the last. He guessed it was a place name but couldn't make sense of it.

Would you recognise the place again?

Jean shrugged. *I would know the house if I was standing outside it. I'm not sure I could take you there.*

And in this house, they looked after you until the baby was born?

She nodded. *I had the baby two weeks later. A doctor came when I first got to the house and then when my time arrived. They were very kind to me. I ate good food, and the maid laundered my clothes. The mistress had ordered gowns and bedding for the baby and I slept in a room just along from the nursery.*

This man. Can you tell me more about him? What age was he? Old? Young?

71

A fair bit older than me, Jean replied.

A similar age to me? Or as old as Mr Sibbald?

She shook her head and flickered her hand back and forth. *In between.*

What did he look like? Robert asked.

Jean indicated that this man had whiskers but no beard or moustache and that his hair was dark brown, a bald patch on the crown. She gestured that he was broad-shouldered and affected a swaggering gait. She puffed out her cheeks.

He was fat? asked Robert.

No, she said, *not fat – burly. He threw his weight about as he moved, as if he thought himself very important.*

And his wife? Can you describe her to me?

About the same age. Very thin, with a pinched face. Her hair is brown with streaks of grey. She looks fragile, like she might snap in two, but she's vicious and full of anger.

Jean's gaze was towards Robert, but she wasn't looking at him. She was staring into the middle distance. As if she were watching something. Robert suspected that there was a scene involving these people that she replayed over and over again.

And were you given the money that had been promised to you?

She nodded again. *All the time I nursed my baby, they paid me two shillings a week. With that, and the pound I had been given, I saved more money than I'd ever had in my life.*

What about Sandy. Where was he, when all this was going on?

He stayed with Jim in Taylor's Close. I went to see him occasionally. They let me go home for a few hours at the end of each week. I delivered some money to Jim for Sandy's keep. Jim was working at the docks now and then and the women in the close looked out for Sandy while he was gone.

Did these women know where you were and what you were doing?

They knew the bare bones of the story. That I was giving my baby to a wealthy couple, but the man made us promise not to tell anyone who they were. A look of sudden recollection passed over Jean's face. *Jim knows their name. He asked for directions at a house when he accompanied me that first day. I had to rest, and he spoke to a wifie who was standing in a doorway.*

Robert's eyes flashed. *So, if I can find Jim Donnelly, do you think he might remember their name?*

I'm sure he would.

The last strands of daylight had begun to weave their way through the bars at the cell window. Jean's face was pale and tired.

I have so many questions, Robert said. *Can you carry on?*

I should like to sleep for a while. Would that be allowed?

Robert nodded reluctantly. *Of course.* He desperately wanted to keep going but they were both weary. Better to rest and return to it the following week.

Once, in London, he had visited Braidwood's school and gone on a trip to Kensington, where one of the patrons showed him what he had referred to as 'a dissection'. It was a wooden map of the British Isles that had been cut into many pieces, along the lines of the various counties. When the pieces were scattered, the game was to fit them back together again. The man who owned it had been a tutor to the sons of George III and this was a memento of that time – he had used it to teach the royal princes their geography. It was an expensive toy but a fascinating one, Robert recalled. On his return to Edinburgh, he and Maggie had experimented with making one of their own by copying a map from an atlas and then cutting it into sections.

Before today, Jean's story had been a similar puzzle, but

he was beginning to make it fit together. He had manoeuvred some of the components into the correct places and was now sorting through the stray pieces, hovering over them, wondering where they might fit. He had a feeling of surety, that it was possible to complete this puzzle and that he was the man to do it.

He stood up. Stretched again to awaken his limbs.

15

~ Saturday, 11 January 1817:
Partickhill Road, Glasgow ~

By the time they reached the steep approach to Partickhill it was getting on for midday. Strands of Jean's hair were stuck to her forehead and her face was red with the effort of the journey.

She carried a small canvas bag containing a change of linen, some hairpins, a comb and a few coins. A low wall ran along the side of a blacksmith's yard and she sat down on it, dismayed at the hill in front of her and with no real idea of the miles she had already walked and how far she still had to go. They had been on the road for over an hour, and she was hungry and thirsty.

Jim continued walking for a few yards before he realised that Jean was no longer immediately behind him and, resentfully, he retraced his steps to join her outside the blacksmith's. He idled nearby while Jean took a jug of water out of the bag, unstoppered it and drank some down. She leant forward, elbows on her knees, palms circling her temples. The child was pushing against her bladder and she desperately needed to piss. Her head was pounding, and she felt shivery, despite the fine day.

She looked at Jim, but he avoided her gaze. He pointed the toe of his boot at the stone wall, kicked at the scraps of moss rooted between the stones. As each clod loosened, he pushed it down and ground it into the dirt road. Jean considered this a pointless act. Jim had pulled down the brim of his hat against the sun and it was ragged and smeared with smuts. He had a black look about him that Jean couldn't be fashed with. She was the one who was suffering to get them out of the hole they'd made for themselves. Yet here he was, acting like she was abandoning him. Like a child throwing a toy to the ground in temper.

They had set off that forenoon from Taylor's Close, leaving Sandy with the wife at the close mouth. She was an old gossip and gey fond of a drink, but she looked after a lot of the local children and she was cheap. Sandy would be safe enough until Jim got back. Jean had tried to make-believe she was just away for the day and would see him again soon. It was easier that way.

They had walked along the north bank of the Clyde, where the Broomielaw's bustle gave way to cottages and gardens. The insects buzzing here were butterflies and bees, not the fat fruit-flies swarming over the city middens. They'd passed the bleachfields at Kelvinhaugh and walked until they reached the spot where the Clyde met the River Kelvin. There, a small wooden bridge took them into Partick. When they had both walked a little further, Jim had asked a couple of men standing on a street corner if they were on the right road for Partickhill and they nodded and pointed them north-west, up the brae. The people here were taller and fairer than in the city, a great many of them hailing from the Highlands having been displaced from their homes, first by sheep farming and then by poverty. Jim said they spoke with an accent a bit like his own Irish and Jean supposed they spoke the Gaelic of her own family in Islay. After a short while, they had turned off the main road onto a wide path. Here, a few buildings dotted the landscape, but it was mostly open grass with rough paths between the houses. Stone walls and hedges marked the boundaries between them.

A woman with two children came out of the blacksmith's yard and looked at them both curiously. She couldn't help but notice that Jean was heavily pregnant.

Jean looked up at her.

'Are you alright, hen?' she asked.

'She's fine, missus,' said Jim. 'She's deaf, mind, she cannae hear you.'

The two children stared at Jean, as if searching for visible proof of her affliction.

'Where are you bound?' asked the woman.

'To the house that belongs to McDougall,' said Jim. 'He has one of the shipyards nearby.'

'Aye, I know it. It's no far. It's a bit of a trauchle to get to the top but you'll be there in no time, tell her. She looks like she's gey far on to be traipsing all ower the place.'

'Thanks, missus,' said Jim. He crouched down by Jean. *This woman says we've not far to go.*

Jean smiled at the woman and her children and gathered her paltry belongings together. She pushed herself back up to a standing position and resumed walking. Jim walked beside her, but they didn't speak to each other. Bitterness emanated from him like slime trailing from a slug. The path was wide and they each cleaved to the opposite side. The wooden soles of Jean's boots were completely worn down in places and sharp points of gravel kept jutting into her feet.

At the top of the hill, a thick boundary wall ran the length of the road to the left and Jim indicated that they should follow its course. According to his instructions, Charles McDougall's house was immediately adjacent to the far end of this old wall. Sure enough, when they had followed the road for a few minutes, a red sandstone villa came into view. It was a square-built house with a doorway in the centre and two storeys with rectangular panelled windows on either side. A path led to the front door and another in the direction of what looked like wooden stables or outbuildings.

Jim hesitated, his previous bullish manner replaced with uncertainty.

Will I come with you? he asked.

Jean looked at him as if he were stupid. *They won't want that.*

A flicker of anger surfaced but he reined himself in and looked down at his feet.

Oh, Christ, he's going to cry, thought Jean.

She took hold of his arm.

Look after Sandy, will you, please?

He sighed and brought his closed hand to his mouth before touching his lips with his index finger. As he brought his hand down, he opened it and rested it on the open palm of his other hand.

I promise. Will you be alright?

She smiled weakly. *Safer to give birth here than in your lodgings. They've got me a doctor. A maid to clear up after me and a cook to make my meals. I'll be better looked after than I've ever been.*

And after?

They'll want me here for a while. To feed the baby.

When will I see you again?

I don't know. It depends when the baby arrives. They won't want me wandering off until they get their hands on it.

Jim grabbed at some trails of ivy that dreeped over the wall, wound them around his fist and pulled, ripping out more than he had intended.

'Fucksake,' he said, untangling the strands and casting them on the ground.

Jean watched him and started laughing. He glared at her.

Fuck are you laughing at?

You. Jean pointed right at him, shaking her head as if he were a madman.

She pulled him towards her and brushed his cheek. Jim's chin was covered with days-old stubble. His dark hair was long and greasy strands curled outwards beneath his ridiculous hat, but his eyes were the clearest blue and his lashes leapt out from them like black sparks. His foul mood and childish temper didn't solve anything, but she understood it.

He couldn't reach into his pocket and produce money that didn't exist and, if there was no money, there could be no baby. These people – the McDougalls – had plenty of money and they wanted a baby. Jean had a baby that she could not provide for. There was little else to be done. Jim felt like he had nothing to offer.

Back home, in Donegal, there was no money either, but a baby would have been welcomed and looked after by his family. Here, for all the people that teemed through the streets and lived and worked cheek by jowl, there was not a one who could help them.

I could come back in a few days, he said, *see if you're alright?*

Jean nodded. *Yes, you wait here. Same time next week. I'll come outside and meet you.*

What if the baby comes before that?

I'll send word to you, she said. *At the Anchor?*

Jim nodded. *We'll raise a toast to the wee man.*

Might be a girl.

Aye, so it might. We'll raise a toast if that's the case, too.

79

A pause. They both knew they should part – they had reached their destination and there was no more to be said – but were reluctant to do so.

Finally, Jean kissed his cheek and walked away.

16

≈ Saturday, 1 March 1817:
Adam Square, Edinburgh ≈

Lord Succoth studied his fingernails, idly pushing back the cuticles as he pondered what Robert had just told him.

'It sounds gey convoluted to me, Kinniburgh,' His Lordship announced. 'Is it not more likely that the panel is covering up for her own or even this Irishman's crime by inventing these so-called adoptive parents?'

Succoth walked over to the fireplace and emptied his pipe into the grate. He reached up to the mantelpiece, opened a polished smoking cabinet and took out a ceramic dish in which he stored his tobacco.

As he turned, his steely grey eyes fixed on Robert. 'Why on earth would a well-to-do couple want to take a baby off a deaf hoor and a papist? It doesn't make much sense. I think Jean Campbell is spinning you a line.'

'I can't deny it's possible that she is, Your Lordship,' said Robert, 'but her conduct, as well as the story itself, has the ring of truth about it. Barren women have been known to do desperate things and husbands are prone to protecting their wives and their own reputations.'

Lord Succoth raised an eyebrow. Robert formed the impression that any discussion of the domestic was frowned upon by His Lordship. A trim, fit man for his age, Succoth was always tidily groomed and impeccably dressed. He seemed to view his cases and those caught up in them as no more than black and white; chess pieces moving around a board in a preordained pattern, rather than human beings navigating the messiness of their relationships and environment.

Succoth sat down in his winged armchair and began to fill his pipe.

'Do you envisage a return to the Tolbooth on Monday morning?'

'With your permission, sir. I'd like to interview the prisoner again. I believe I now have her confidence and she assures me that she has more to tell.'

'That's all very well, Kinniburgh, but could she not simply give you the names of the couple so that an investigation as to the veracity of her claims might take place?'

'Well, I'd like to visit Glasgow to do that if I can, sir. That's why I wish to speak to her further. She can't give me the names of these people because she doesn't know them.'

Succoth peered at Robert incredulously.

'What kind of daupit creature would go to live with folk without knowing their names? Let alone hand over her own child to them?'

'A deaf woman who is also illiterate, sir,' Robert replied. 'If one is not able to hear someone's name and can neither read it nor spell it, then there's not much use to be had from that name. I can believe that might have been Jean Campbell's experience.'

'Well, it sounds like a rum deal to me, but I'll take your word for it. Be sure of your facts before you go haring off to Glasgow, though. I'm only willing to pay for so much in relation to this woman's case.'

Succoth closed his tobacco case and set it down on the arm of his chair. He cradled the bowl of his pipe in his palm. With his other hand, he reached into the pocket of his waistcoat for his watch and shifted in his seat, as if to convey that the audience granted Robert was coming to a close.

17

~ *Monday, 3 March 1817:*
The Tontine Hotel, Glasgow ~

Robert was ensconced in a firmly upholstered armchair in a corner of a large, oval room. A pewter coffee pot was positioned in the centre of a mahogany side table, but he balanced his cup and saucer in his lap. It was almost nine o'clock, but the ground floor piazza was still busy. Full of guests and locals alike.

It had been the back of seven in the evening when Robert alighted from a stagecoach at the Trongate. After his dismissal from Lord Succoth's presence on Saturday evening, Archibald Gibson, with the minimum of fuss, had arranged his travel and furnished him with sufficient monies to cover accommodation and any other reasonable expenses he might incur.

Robert's own arrangements at Chessels Court had been less satisfactory. After showing his face at church, he had flouted the Sabbath by attending to the papers that had piled up on his desk over the last few days. All the while avoiding Maggie's sideways glances that appraised and found him wanting.

On his arrival at the Trongate, he had been grateful to get out of the cramped confines of the coach. It had left Edinburgh at twenty past seven that morning and his entire body now felt compressed and constricted. The coach had stopped only twice during the twelve-hour journey, first at Uphall and then at Kirk of Shotts. At both places, the coachmen changed their horses, and the few passengers went within to have something to eat and drink before resuming their travels.

He waited in the rain beside a statue of King William and, once he had collected his small leather bag from the coachman, presented himself in the reception area of the hotel. Alone in his room, he'd stretched out on the soft mattress of the large bed and rested for half an hour before washing and coming down to eat supper and wait for Angus Buchanan to arrive.

Archibald Gibson had sent word to the Reverend Buchanan by messenger, introducing Robert and asking if they might meet to discuss the Jean Campbell case. Robert had plans to seek out some of the players in the drama and he suspected the clergyman might be a good man to provide the relevant connections and perhaps offer some insights of his own.

Robert had never seen anything quite like the Tontine. Built in the Italian style, a series of decorated arches formed the ground floor, with the hotel and various municipal facilities on the storeys above. Each arch was decorated with the face of a different grotesque, which leered down as one entered the building. Weary from his travels, Robert found their unfamiliar aspects more menacing than perhaps he would have done in the light of day.

~

The west coast accents in the room took him back to his youth. His childhood home at Kirkintilloch was only a few miles north-east of the city but he had visited Glasgow only a handful of times. He remembered a trip taken with his father along the Monklands Canal. Robert couldn't have been more than ten years old. His father travelling to meet some merchant in the city.

They'd boarded a canal boat in Kirkintilloch and Robert recalled the sudden lurch of the boat as he'd stepped onto the deck, a nervous laugh as his father grabbed his arm to steady him. They'd hunkered down together, their backs against piles of cargo, legs stretched out on the wooden boards. A skein of geese flew overhead, and Robert had watched as they cut effortlessly through a cloudless sky. Where the canal widened, the scow ploughed confidently through the water and when it narrowed again, the boatman had performed a side-to-side dance that levered them safely away from the canal walls. Robert had stuck his hand out and let the reeds twist in his fingers, releasing hosts of tiny insects whose wings sparked bright blue.

'What are they, Da?'

'That's dragonflies, I think, son,' his father had answered. 'They look like they're lit up from the inside, don't they?'

Dragonflies. Flies that were also dragons. Tiny flying dragons.

At intervals they'd slowed down, almost to a halt, while the horse guided them under a bridge. The motion of the water and the warmth of the day had eased young Robert into a slumber and when he awoke, he found that the canal had opened out and the boatman was busy steering them through a huge basin and into another narrower branch of water. With a start, Robert had realised he was alone. He'd scrambled to his feet, but his father was only standing on the bank, holding the cuddie's reins, and waiting for the scow to settle into the right channel and resume their journey.

Eventually they'd reached a wharf, high above Glasgow, where the boatman got out and wound a length of thick rope around an iron bollard. Robert and his father had bid the man goodbye and, carrying two bags apiece, walked gingerly down a steep set of wooden steps to the road below. They'd tramped a half mile or so past large houses and gardens until the buildings grew denser and the people more numerous.

At a public house called the Swan, his father had hailed an acquaintance and ordered whiskies for them both and a small beer for Robert. Robert had taken his drink into the street and begun eating the bread and cheese his mother had packed for him. There were lots of people going about their business, carters loading and unloading, adjusting the nosebags on their horses or stopping to let the beasts drink from a well at the side of the road. There was a row of shops on the opposite side of the road from the Swan: a baker; a milliner; and a tobacconist. The young women in the baker's shop wore impossibly white starched aprons and their hair was scraped back beneath patterned bonnets. In the milliner's, a doll-like woman reached into the window and held a hat aloft. Men in expensive-looking clothes and tall hats formed a steady stream in and out of the tobacconists.

~

'Mr Kinniburgh?'

Robert was shaken from his reverie by a small, smiling man wearing a clergyman's collar.

'Reverend Buchanan? Excuse me, I was away in a world of my own. Do join me, sir.' Robert gestured to the minister to sit down opposite him and asked if he would like a drink.

'Och, that's very kind of you. I don't go in for this coffee and what have you, but I'll take a small whisky if they have one.'

Robert ordered a whisky for the Reverend Buchanan and one for himself. They exchanged a few pleasantries about the comfort of the coffee rooms and the convenient location of the hotel.

When the drinks arrived, Buchanan asked, 'And how is our Jean, Mr Kinniburgh?'

'Distressed, but she's as well as can be expected,' replied Robert, 'under the circumstances. She's not been ill-treated and has been telling me something of her story, but I confess I am impeded in gathering the details that might help make her case. As I mentioned in my letter, she has furnished me with fragments about her life in Glasgow and I hoped it would help me to elicit more from her by visiting the people and places she speaks of. I believe you have known her for some time?'

The minister nodded. 'Jean has been attending our society for a fair few years now. The deaf in the city, not to mention myself and my wife, are very fond of her. We were all shocked to hear that she had been arrested and when we discovered the charge was the murder of a baby, well, that seems so unlike our Jean to be quite unbelievable, Mr Kinniburgh.'

'You would describe Jean as a respectable woman, Mr Buchanan?'

'Yes.'

'Despite her domestic arrangements and having had two illegitimate children?'

'Well, perhaps not respectable,' the minister replied, ruefully. 'But I would certainly describe Jean Campbell as a good woman, someone I would trust.'

'Did you know she was pregnant?'

'I heard that, yes. What I knew was that she was living with a chap called Donnelly and had got herself in trouble. She was still coming to society meetings up until the end of last summer and then a few weeks went by when no one heard anything of her. We assumed that she'd started to show and was embarrassed to come along. No one likes to be the centre of gossip, do they?'

Robert looked puzzled. 'And none of you thought to make sure she was alright? Excuse my directness, but if Jean was a valued member of your community, would you not seek her out?'

'I wish I had, Mr Kinniburgh, but it was not quite as easy as you might think.'

'What do you mean?' Robert asked.

The minister sighed. 'If Jean had still been living with her aunt and uncle, we would have known where to go to enquire as to her welfare. The rumour was that she was living in the Saltmarket. It's a rough place. Not somewhere you wander about unless you need to.'

Robert nodded.

'It wasn't that we forgot about Jean, Mr Kinniburgh. Many of the congregation were puzzled and concerned about her. Some suspected, in light of her trouble, she'd gone back to her people in the islands.'

'But she hadn't, had she?' said Robert.

The minister sighed. 'It would appear not, Mr Kinniburgh.'

'Jean told me that she wasn't in the Saltmarket with Donnelly. Not all that time, at any rate,' said Robert. 'She said a well-to-do couple gave her board and lodging, offered to adopt her baby. For a price.'

The Reverend Buchanan looked at Robert in disbelief.

'Jean says she met the man at your church.'

18

~ Saturday, 21 September 1816:
Partickhill Road, Glasgow ~

In the kitchen, Martha Sproull began gathering her bits and pieces to take upstairs. She was to turn out the mistress's bedroom. She needed dusters and blacking paste and had still to make up a bowl of oil and vinegar polish. The job hadn't been on today's list of chores, but Mrs Drysdale suggested she seize this unexpected opportunity to clean and air the room.

Mrs McDougall had been allowed outside for the first time in weeks and was currently propped up with cushions in a wicker chair in the garden, a shawl wrapped around her shoulders. Martha had taken a cup of beef tea on a tray and fetched the mistress's book for her, but Mrs McDougall had not reached for either and had simply gazed distractedly at her fingers as they laced and unlaced in her lap.

'Wabbit, so she is,' pronounced Mrs Drysdale, looking out at Euphemia McDougall from the narrow scullery window. 'The doctor's gave her that many pills and potions, she disnae have a clue what day it is.'

Mrs Drysdale continued her surveillance as she measured flour on the scales and sieved it into an earthenware bowl. The cook placed it on a tray, along with some yeast, and carried her cargo back into the kitchen, where she poured some water from a pitcher into the mixture, took up her wooden spoon and began beating with a vengeance.

'That many weans she's lost. I widnae wish that on

anybody. That basturt should stop tormenting the poor woman.'

'What do you mean, tormenting her?' Martha asked.

The cook shrugged off Martha's question.

'I should haud my wheest, hen,' said Mrs Drysdale, turning the bread mix out of her bowl onto the floured wooden table.

Martha watched the cook working, marvelling at the strength in Mrs Drysdale's scrawny arms. Every bit of sinew and muscle in operation, the slight flap of aged skin escaping from her tightly rolled sleeves. Mrs Drysdale was in her late sixties, her skin lined and weather-beaten, but she could still work from early morning to late at night, without tiring or complaining. A greater contrast to the mistress, with her buttermilk skin smoothed over her mind's torment, Martha couldn't imagine.

As a rule, Mrs Drysdale worked at the McDougalls' six mornings a week, preparing meals, overseeing the vegetable garden and buying supplies from the local market. She was a woman who, generally, held no truck with weakness. And yet Martha had noticed on more than one occasion that the cook often took pains to make sure Euphemia McDougall was catered for.

The older woman lived close by Martha's parents in the cottages on Castlebank Street, near Merkland's sawmills. Mr Drysdale had been employed in the sawmill until a few years ago but was now an invalid, confined at home. Martha had known them all her life and Mrs Drysdale had mentioned her name when the McDougalls were looking for a new domestic. The cook's full name was Donaldina Drysdale and, as a child, Martha had known her as Ina. But in the big house in Partickhill, she was always sure to address her as Mrs Drysdale.

~

Martha hummed a tune as she blackened the grate in the mistress's bedroom. She was firmly of the opinion that there was no point everybody going around looking like they were chewing wasps. Still, that was Presbyterians for you, as Martha's father often said. Cultivators of the pursed lip and disapproving shudder.

She had opened the sash and case windows as far as she could, and a crisp breeze was hurling its way into the mistress's bedroom, sweeping out the smell of sickness from hidden corners as Martha scrubbed the surfaces clean.

By the time she rose to her feet, her fingers were black and a filthy mix of dust and stoor was packed tight around her short nails. She caught sight of herself in the huge mirror suspended over the mantelpiece. A dark curl had escaped from her cap and she pushed it back, leaving a smear of coal dust across one cheekbone. She winked and blew her reflection a kiss.

19

~ Saturday, 21 September 1816:
Partickhill Road, Glasgow ~

Charles paused at the back door and appraised his wife. Against the cheerful greens and reds of rosehips and rowan berries, she looked spectral, like a phantom from a ghost story. She wore a shapeless, pale-coloured dress and her shoulders were covered with a dark green and yellow paisley shawl. Her brown hair had been scraped back and pinned into a bun at the nape of her neck.

It was a warm day and Charles had come from a morning at the dockyard. He had climbed up to Partickhill in a hurry and now stood in his shirtsleeves and heavy trousers surveying the topography of his home life. Lines of sweat appeared at his temples. He held in his hand a draught from the doctor and a glass of Solomon's Cordial Balm.

Charles crossed the grassy patch of garden and hunkered down in front of Euphemia. He placed the glass and packet on a three-legged stool that served as a side table and leant his hand on the arm of his wife's chair.

'I've brought your medicine, dear. Would you like me to mix it in your cordial?'

Euphemia stared at him. A glassy-eyed gaze that spoke of absence and a peculiar strain of revulsion. The source of this revulsion was a mystery to Charles. Sometimes he thought it was he who disgusted her. Other times he suspected she hated herself. Perhaps it was a combination of the two. Perhaps there had been a time when he would have been interested in the answer.

She remained silent. Charles tried another tack.

'I could go back to the kitchen and get a glass of water as well. Would you prefer that?'

He hauled himself up and positioned the other wicker chair to face his wife. He sat down.

'Euphemia?'

'Yes?'

Euphemia suddenly snapped into life, focusing on him with a birdlike alertness. In the normal course of things, Charles was not an empathetic man, but even he could sense that her distaste had not dissipated and was merely suspended under a deceptively still surface.

'I was talking about your medicine. You should take it.'

Euphemia's eyes flicked towards the glass and the doctor's draught and flicked back to Charles.

'Oh, I see. Do you?'

'Dr Wilson said it would help, dear.'

Euphemia sniffed and shook her head.

'Surely you don't think a sleeve of powder and some quack's tonic will cure me, do you, Charles?'

Charles sighed. 'It might make you feel better.'

Euphemia rolled her words like little bullets in her mouth and spat them out at him.

'Even you can't be that stupid, Charles.'

'That's enough, Euphemia,' Charles said wearily.

Euphemia began to worry at her fingers. She manipulated the knuckle of her thumb back and forth, back and forth, until it clicked and cracked. A small enough sound in itself, it ricocheted around the festering atmosphere between them. It was intrusive, like listening to the incessant barking of a dog left locked up for the day.

'Well,' she said, shrugging 'if Dr Wilson and the

so-called-doctor Solomon are responsible for my care, I might as well relinquish all hope now.'

'Dr Wilson is a respected physician, dear. He's called upon by some of the best families in the city. I'm sure he has your best interests at heart.'

Euphemia laughed.

'Dr Wilson is a chronic inebriate, *dear*. I'm sure that what is closest to his heart is his next drink. And, as for Dr Solomon of Liverpool, he claims his watery liquid is able to do everything except raise the dead. Preposterous. Only an idiot would be taken in by that charlatan.'

Charles looked at her as if she were an imbecile.

'The testimonials for his Gilead cure speak for themselves.'

Euphemia smiled and shook her head.

'For a man of business, Charles, you really are spectacularly naive. Do you honestly believe that those letters in the newspaper advertisements and his badly written book are anything other than concoctions of Dr Solomon himself? He's not even a real doctor. Apparently, he started off as a boot polish salesman in Newcastle.'

'What difference does that make?' Charles snapped.

'All the difference in the world.'

Euphemia's scorn was like a red rag to a bull. As usual, Charles felt a compunction to defend the honour of those born to less privilege than his lady wife.

'So, it's beyond the bounds of possibility that a boot polish salesman could do anything of note?'

Euphemia affected consideration of this notion for a few moments.

'It's highly unlikely, yes.'

'I'm an engineer, Euphemia. I started off the son of a farm labourer. It's not completely unheard of for talent to rise above a man's origins.'

'An engineer? I believe you had a trade. Joinery, wasn't

it? Engineer is a title you acquired for yourself, is it not? Much like the esteemed Dr Solomon.'

At the beginning of every conversation with her husband, Euphemia resolved to keep her dignity, withhold from him the satisfaction of seeing any more of her distress. Invariably, however, she failed. She could not resist an opportunity to patronise him, to wound Charles in retaliation for the constant hurt he caused her.

His oxters were damp, and Charles could feel his anger rising.

'Watch your tongue, lady,' he growled. 'I worked hard to get where I am, and you benefit from my efforts and should show some gratitude.'

Euphemia looked him up and down.

'You got where you are on the back of my father's money.'

'Don't you dare speak to me like that in my own house.'

'Or what?' she asked. 'What will you do if I don't behave? Put me away? Stop paying me attention? That would be a blessed relief.'

Euphemia's face coloured and she cursed herself for giving way to the surfeit of emotion that collected inside her. It was self-defeating, to begin an argument with Charles. Yet she could not stop. Her breathing became more ragged as she fought back the tableau of obscene images that crowded her mind.

'I want no more of your filthy seed in me and no more of your feeble babies that just die and die and die.' She spat the words at him.

Charles could feel a familiar rage gather within him. He wanted to knock her into next week. He could hear a clattering of pans from the kitchen and the sound of Mrs Drysdale's tuneless singing, so he held his fury in, but he would have liked to crack Euphemia's jaw for her. To pull her down by the hair and hit her until she promised to show him the respect that he was due.

As they lapsed into silence once more, he played out his fantasy, imagined her lying beneath him, scrabbling to get clear, while he decided the best way to bring her to heel.

Charles had had enough of her carrying on. He got up from the chair, poured the contents of Wilson's brown paper package into the glass of liquid and handed it to his wife.

'Take your medicine, Euphemia. Then I'll get Martha to help you back to bed.'

Euphemia drank it down in two gulps, some of it escaping the corners of her mouth and running down her chin. She brought her hand up to her face and wiped it away. She looked as though she might cry.

Charles smirked.

'Good girl. Now, if you continue to behave yourself, you may come down for dinner later.'

20

～ Saturday, 21 September 1816:
Partickhill Road, Glasgow ～

Euphemia's fingers felt numb and useless as she tried to fasten the ribbon of her bedjacket. She had sent Martha downstairs and insisted on getting into bed by herself. The sleeping draught had made her groggy and rendered her incapable of completing the most mundane of tasks. Her earlier anger had dissipated, but that gave her no relief.

Before her marriage, Euphemia was not wholly ignorant of the intimacies that occurred between husband and wife. However, the little she knew of the theory ill - prepared her for the horror of the practice. She had already been thirty-two when she met Charles, and just over a year older than that on the day of her wedding.

Her mother had taken her aside and told her that Charles would expect his due as a husband. It was Euphemia's duty to bear it; the act would get easier as time went by and she settled down to married life.

Euphemia found that she could not bear it. The physical act itself was unpleasant and painful at first, but she had grown used to that. What she could not reconcile herself to was that it left her, each time, with a sense of shame so deep she could barely articulate it to herself. That her husband's expression, after the fact, was perpetually one of relief rather than ecstasy served only to compound her wretchedness.

When she had accepted Charles's marriage proposal,

she had no illusions that he might covet her, but she had harboured hopes that they might have a pleasant enough union of convenience, that she might prove to be his help-meet and he, her protector. It took only a little time for her to be disabused of these notions.

It was a cruel irony that, even under such loveless circum-stances, Euphemia had no difficulty becoming pregnant. But with each failed attempt at carrying a child to full term, the whole rigmarole would have to begin anew.

She herself had been an only child, welcomed and indulged. An older brother and sister having both died in infancy, her father and mother were desperately careful of their surviving progeny. Euphemia was sickly as a baby and grew up to be pale and wan, intellectually sharp but not possessed of those most prized attributes – the ability to smile sweetly and converse effortlessly at the most tire-some of gatherings and amongst the dullest of people. Her parents did not stint on her upbringing; she had been weaned and schooled and trundled around Glaswegian society as bait while they searched for a suitable husband for her. After more than ten years when she had been all but swallowed up by spinsterhood, her parents' fortitude had gradually failed, and the small family became a resigned and somewhat resentful trio in a pretty townhouse in Virginia Street. Until the day that her father was called upon by an engineer who wished to engage a man to see to his accounts.

21

~ Saturday, 21 September 1816:
Partickhill Road, Glasgow ~

Charles took up his penknife and sharpened the quill that lay on his desk. He opened the top of the inkwell and filled the nib, tapping out some excess ink in readiness for his task.

He was completing his purchase ledger for the previous month, as he always did, by making permanent those transactions that he was prepared to admit to. He kept a list of balances with his true creditors in pencil in a private pocketbook. A tally of secrets that he did not intend to share with his wife or her father.

Charles's left hand smoothed the sheet of paper in the ledger, while his right hand scratched and composed his latest fiction.

~

Charles had first met his future father-in-law at a large firm of chartered accountants who kept their offices in a suite of rooms off St Vincent Street. Hector Rintoul was a senior man, in charge of a team of bookkeepers, loss-adjustors and insurers. Charles had set up as a shipping engineer the previous summer and business had been brisk, going from strength to strength over the first few months. The initial business was so successful, in fact, that the small yard he leased out at Finnieston proved to be wholly unsuitable for meeting the contracts he had acquired.

By the time Charles met Hector Rintoul, he had moved production to a larger yard near Partick. His staff were working all out to meet their obligations, but the administration of his business was in complete chaos. At a social event at the Merchants' Hall, an acquaintance had commiserated with him and recommended that he employ someone to keep an eye on his books.

Like many self-made men, Charles was reluctant to seek advice on work of any kind. He did not trust anyone else to have his best interests at heart and, if he was completely honest, there were elements of his business practice that he preferred to keep to himself. However, he'd arranged a meeting with Rintoul and endeavoured to put his best foot forward.

Commercial offices in the city relied on industries to keep them busy, but there was something about their polished and panelled interiors that made Charles acutely uncomfortable. On the one hand, he felt that he was a man of means, doing the firm a favour by deigning to engage them. On the other, he felt compelled to tug at his forelock and apologise for his dirty boots.

Charles had arrived at Hector Rintoul's office early on a Friday morning. A clerk bade him sit in an antechamber on a backless bench that ran the length of one side of the room. There was a very narrow window that stretched from halfway down the exterior wall almost to the floor and looked out onto the street. Charles couldn't understand its design. It was as if the building had been subdivided in a rather haphazard way. The room was bare and devoid of reading matter of any kind, so Charles had shuffled along the bench to a vantage point that allowed him to look outside. The window looked out onto a narrow lane where mean side entrances spilled out onto cobbles and middens had piled up.

It was a gloomy scene. Charles had noticed an old man, well-dressed but swaying slightly, staggering into the middle of the lane and watched as two young men, hatted but barefoot, emerged from a doorway.

The young men glanced about them and approached the older man. In a heartbeat, they had their arms around his shoulders and inside his pockets. From a distance, Charles could not hear what they were saying, but he could guess at the gammon in their language by the snide looks each gave the other while whispering support and succour in the older man's ear.

The younger men had diverged, full of braggadocio now that a fat wallet lay snug in one of their hands and a weighty pocket watch in another. They became bolder and less solicitous of their mark. The lads had adopted a swagger, jostling the man where before they had held him up. One of them knocked him to the side while making a pretence of putting an arm around his shoulders. The old man had slipped on the grimy surface of the road and tumbled against a pile of manure that had been shovelled into a corner. The young men had laughed, making a game of it to hide their shame. Inexplicably, Charles had felt a pull in his groin and his prick had swelled. He'd reached down to rub himself as the lads made off along the lane and the old man thrashed helplessly amidst the excrement in which he found himself, befuddled as to what had brought him there.

Charles had continued to touch himself, quite openly, through the worsted of his breeches. There was a part of him that was given over to whatever pleasure or release he was taking from the scene and there was another part of him that surveyed both the assault and robbery of the old man and his own behaviour, and could make no sense of either.

~

Charles laid down his quill on a piece of dusting cloth and surveyed the ledger. It was becoming harder to conceal the downturn in business that his yard had lately suffered. It would be even harder to explain to Hector Rintoul once this deception became apparent, as it surely would. Charles had harboured expectations of securing some of the construction work attached to the works on widening the river and improving access to the city. It had not been forthcoming. Despite his attempts to inveigle himself into Glasgow's society, his rise, if it existed at all, had been imperceptible.

The money that had come to him on marrying Euphemia had seemed substantial, at least enough to get his business on a firm foundation. But it had slipped through his fingers, and no more was likely from that source unless he could produce an heir to act as key to the Rintoul coffers.

This was the source of his frustration and Euphemia's distress. If she could carry a child to term, all would be well. And then Charles thought about the woman he had met outside the Deaf Church and to whom, through a rudimentary exchange of words and gestures, he had offered his help.

22

~ Tuesday, 4 March 1817:
Calton, Glasgow ~

Robert navigated his way through the confusion of people and vehicles that traversed the streets around the Trongate. He had risen early and breakfasted at the hotel and was now heading eastwards to meet Angus Buchanan at his church.

Buchanan had suggested that he join him to talk further about Jean's life in Glasgow. He had also offered to furnish Robert with a map and directions that might lead him to discover both the whereabouts of the errant Jim Donnelly and the places that Jean had been frequenting in the weeks leading up to the incident on the Old Bridge.

The previous evening, Buchanan had been taken aback at Jean's tale of her encounter with a couple who meant to procure her baby. He had professed that it was not something that he had been a party to, and he was at a loss as to who these people might be. He had told Robert that he had ministered in the city for many years and his deaf church had become something of a curiosity for the hearing as well as a refuge for the deaf. A great number of people came through his doors for one reason and another.

The crush of Glasgow's citizens thinned out a little as Robert made his way towards the Calton. It was the back of eight and the area's workers were already busy at their occupations. Here, weavers' cottages and small industries huddled together in a jumble of buildings that had been added to as the city drew in goods and immigrants from all over the globe.

With little heed for planning or coordination, makeshift communities had grown up, intersecting with those of the original city or filling up patches of available space on its outskirts. Landowners had sold up willingly, tempted by the promise of a healthy profit. A stubborn few held on to their substantial estates, and elegant villas and rigidly planted gardens now sat incongruously amidst the upheaval around them.

The day was proving unseasonably mild, so Robert stopped for a minute to take off his greatcoat and tuck it around the strap of the leather bag he was carrying. This held his notebook and pencil as well as some literature about the school that he had brought with him, which he intended to circulate to any interested parties he might meet while in the city.

Just recently, Robert had held a presentation in Edinburgh, exhibiting his teaching methods in an attempt to raise additional funds for the school. In this venture he had involved a number of his pupils, who had quite surpassed themselves in demonstrating their prowess in all manner of academic pursuits. The presentation had been surprisingly lucrative and had also led to increased enquiries from the families of deaf children as to whether their offspring might benefit from attending the Deaf and Dumb Institution.

Afterwards, Margaret had suggested that he might travel to other places, in order to spread the word about the school and attract additional pupils and benefactors. To this end, he had recently prepared a short summary of his methods, along with an invitation to write to him and arrange an event. When he had taken the text to Blackwell's, the printer had encouraged him to make his pamphlet attractive and eye-catching by means of some kind of illustration. Having no artistic ability, Robert had prevailed upon Margaret to help him and she had drawn a simple pen and ink sketch of the school buildings in Chessels Court. Robert was pleased with the result and had brought a bundle of these pamphlets with him to Glasgow. It was not his primary focus, but Margaret had persuaded him that it wouldn't hurt to have a few to hand.

As Robert adjusted his bag and righted himself, he looked beyond the stone wall in front of him and into a meadow surrounded by evergreen trees. Purple and yellow crocuses clustered the grass, bathed by the morning sun. The scene was such a contrast to the mean interior of the Edinburgh Tolbooth and the human stew of Glasgow. Robert felt suddenly optimistic that he would find some answers here that might help Jean Campbell.

~

Robert let the brass knocker fall on the green paint of the door. The house where the Buchanans lived was adjacent to their church and was a simple two-storey structure that, although plain, looked a deal fresher than the ramshackle cottages that surrounded it. Angus Buchanan opened the door and beckoned Robert inside. The minister, his shirt-sleeves rolled up to the elbows under a waistcoat and again sporting his black shirt and clerical collar, greeted his visitor warmly.

'Come away in, Mr Kinniburgh,' he said.

'Call me Robert, please.'

Angus nodded enthusiastically. 'Aye, let's not stand on ceremony. You can call me Angus.' He divested Robert of his hat and coat, hanging them on one of a row of hooks in the hallway. He steered Robert through to a small parlour where a fair-haired woman in her late fifties and a rangy young man were readying themselves to take tea at a round table.

Angus undertook to make the introductions to his wife, Catriona, and David, his son. Robert fished his notebook and pencil from his bag and noted their names. David Buchanan signed to indicate that he understood Robert so far and made it known that he was able to lip-read to some extent.

Would it help if I moved opposite you? Robert offered.

David nodded.

When they were all settled, Robert faced David and said, *I will try to make myself clear, but if I forget myself, please call me to order again. It is important to me that all of you understand my questions.*

David nodded. *I can understand you fine, so far. You can't be much worse than my mother, who waves her hands all over the place like she's guiding a ship into shore.* The young man laughed.

Angus smiled at this, shaking his fist in mock approbation at his son. Mrs Buchanan looked bemused for a second, belatedly cottoning on that David was making fun of her.

She adopted a stern expression, and both signed and spoke back to him. *That's a terrible way to talk about your own mother. If you're not careful, I'll not let you have a scone when they're ready.*

Ah, thought Robert, that's what the glorious smell creeping from the kitchen was. He turned to David once again.

Do you use signs outside your own home?

Yes, I can. David nodded. *But only with those that have some signing in common with me. With my parents and my employer and some deaf friends. Outside of that, I have to read peoples' expressions and their lips to make sense of what they are saying. I can read, of course. My father taught me.*

'David is well used to communicating with all manner of company, Robert,' Angus interjected. 'He's not backwards in coming forwards if he needs a point clarified. However, let us return to the matter uppermost in all of our minds, the plight of our friend and fellow traveller, Miss Campbell. How can we help you to help her?'

Robert explained Jean's situation as it stood and asked the Buchanans if they could shed any light on what had gone on before she was arrested. They expressed the same mystification as to why she would have thrown the child into the river. All of them shared Angus's previously stated ignorance of where Jean had been in the weeks before she was arrested.

Mrs Buchanan drew her shawl around her and placed her hand on the tabletop, which Robert took as an indication that she had something to say.

'Jean told me she had a way to make sure her baby would be looked after,' Mrs Buchanan said. 'I took it to mean she had in place some kind of plan.'

'Do you know what this plan was?' Robert asked.

'Not really,' she answered. 'Jean mentioned that she had met a man with money who had offered to help her. Everyone knew that she was struggling to look after wee Sandy, never mind another baby, and that Jim Donnelly that she'd taken up with, well, he's not two pennies to rub together.' Mrs Buchanan rolled her eyes. 'To be honest with you, Robert, I didn't set much store by what Jean was saying. People in difficult situations often make claims that are more fantasy than reality. It's a way of coping, I suppose.'

'Do you think this wealthy couple are an invention?' Robert said.

Mrs Buchanan sighed. 'I couldn't say. I'm simply telling you what my impression was at the time. I wish now that I'd paid more attention. It's just that Jean sometimes told stories, made out that her circumstances were better than they were. Pride, I suppose. Nobody likes to be judged, especially by those they call friends, and she was living in sin with a rough papist. She hadn't had much to start with but, still, she'd fallen far.'

Angus took up the story. 'I don't think he's a bad man, that Donnelly fellow. Jean certainly seemed gey fond of him. Just unfortunate that his religion was a problem. It's easier for everyone, I suppose, if like goes with like, but sometimes the heart has other ideas.'

'There's a lot of animosity towards the Irish, Robert,' said Mrs Buchanan, adopting a confidential air. 'They've brought wages down all over the city and the old weavers having to give up their own looms or go cap in hand to the factory bosses for a pittance. It never would have happened if the Irish hadn't cut in and accepted bad conditions.'

David sighed with exasperation. *There's only bad conditions because the factory bosses come up with them in the first place*, he declared. *The Irish are poor and hungry, what do you expect them to do when a wage is offered to them, however small? What would you do, if it was your family who were starving?*

His mother shrugged. She was obviously well used to her son espousing radical views.

'I know it's not the fault of the Irish themselves,' said Angus. 'They're just looking for work, same as everyone else. It's just that they keep to themselves and practise their religion. They make little attempt to bridge the divide.'

It's not the Irish that have made the divide, David said.

Angus made a sign of acquiescence. This was obviously

a bone of contention between them and something he'd rather not debate in the presence of a visitor.

The wind having been taken out of his sails, David turned towards Robert again. *Irish or not, Jean had decided to take up with Jim Donnelly.*

Robert was confused. 'This Donnelly character, he couldn't have been the man with money that Jean was talking about, could he?'

Donnelly doesn't have a pot to piss in, scoffed David. *Excuse my language, but the man's a casual labourer and a drinker to boot. He didn't have enough money to look after himself, never mind a family.*

'I would like to speak to him, nevertheless. Perhaps he might know who this mysterious benefactor of Jean's was?'

Mrs Buchanan seemed unimpressed. 'How could Jean have a benefactor? Who would give her money?'

Jean's a good-looking woman, David said.

Maybe, agreed his mother, *but she's not the type of woman some rich man would marry and take around the town, is she? If someone did that, they'd be wanting something in return.*

Mrs Buchanan turned to Robert. 'They said that Jean was drunk on the bridge, do you think she dropped the baby by accident?'

Robert shook his head. 'She says no. She denies completely that she was drunk.'

Do you believe her? asked David.

I do.

Robert looked at Angus. 'Do you have an address for this man, Jim Donnelly?'

'I believe he lives somewhere around the Saltmarket, but I'm not sure where exactly. I know he drinks in a public house called the Anchor. It might be possible to find him there. I'm not sure you'll find it salubrious. It's certainly not a place to frequent after dark.'

'I'll go there, Angus. Thank you. I can drop into the Anchor this afternoon.'

'But you will stay and eat with us first, Robert?' Mrs Buchanan asked him.

'Please, if I may.'

23

As he made his way towards the Saltmarket, Robert noticed the gait and appearance of the pedestrians he passed become increasingly stooped and haggard. The Calton was a poor, working-class area, no one who lived there had an existence that was anything other than hand-to-mouth, but the Saltmarket was home to some of the most pathetic human specimens that Robert had ever seen.

Men with badly healed scars kept upright only by doorsteps and ingoes; toothless old women engaged in begging for food; feral children, blank-eyed, barefoot and ragged, their skin blue with cold. Despite being forewarned, Robert was disturbed by what he saw. That this level of poverty and despair could exist on such a scale only a few hundred yards from his lodgings at the perjink Tontine Hotel was incomprehensible.

Robert was aware that he stood out in this district and could feel people's eyes alighting on him as he beat a path to the Anchor. His decent clothes and upright demeanour spoke of difference. His confidence shaken, he feared he was a lucrative target for beggars and a providential mark for thieves.

A young woman with a dark, painted mouth accosted him at the corner of the Green. That isn't strictly true, he thought. Not accosted, exactly, but she lurched in front of him, in a beseeching manner. She grabbed a hold of his arm and gestured that he might accompany her into the nearby burial ground. He pulled quickly away, and she stumbled against a low wall, scraping her hand as she reached out to steady herself. He felt a strange mixture of concern and disgust as her face twisted and she spat out a torrent of abuse.

'Ye fuckin gowk. Nae need to push me.'

'I'm sorry,' he said, reaching out a hand to help her up.

He immediately regretted his ingrained politeness as she rose up and continued to berate him. Her speech was slurred and her accent too thick for him to follow closely, but he got the gist. She seemed to be aggrieved that he had turned down her offer of a kneetrembler amongst the dead and was determined to get reparation.

Robert turned and quickened his step, but the woman barrelled along the street beside him.

'Come on. That no worth a couple pennies, pal?' she asked, shoving her grazed hand out in front of Robert's face.

A group of women on the other side of the street turned to watch them, laughing, whether at himself or the unfortunate woman who was buzzing around him like an angry wasp, he wasn't sure.

'See that?' she shouted across to them. 'See the fuckin' state he's left me in?'

Her audience certainly didn't appear concerned or at all inclined to come to the woman's aid.

In panic, Robert fished some small coins out of his pocket and, without examining them, pushed them into the woman's outstretched fist. This financial success seemed to stop her in her tracks and, as she was counting the money, Robert took the opportunity to gather pace and cut round the next corner out of sight. Red-faced and sweating, he dropped his gaze to the street and walked in the direction of the river.

~

The Anchor was, as Angus had suggested, not the most select public house that Robert had ever frequented. It had an entrance but no door as such, just a wooden frame worked into the surrounding heavy stone walls with a couple of rusted hinges hanging useless and limp. A piece of heavy fabric had been pulled across and looped over an iron hook driven into the stone inside the doorway. A faded pattern of blue and green was still discernible on the remaining woollen parts of the fabric – which might have been an old carpet or wall hanging. Robert ducked down under the lintel and edged his way inside.

In the Kirkintilloch of his youth, there had been an established hierarchy of taverns, inns and drinking dens that the denizens of the town seemed to negotiate with ease. Robert's father was a man who would drink beer and spirits on market days in the coaching inns near the town's square. At home, he always had a jug of porter to share with various colleagues and acquaintances if they should happen to drop into his workshop. Robert was sure, however, that his father would never have ventured into the illicit drop houses that operated from the corner of private houses in the vennels and alleyways off the main street. These were places where money changed hands for home-brewed liquor. The town authorities affected a great crusade against these activities, but they had few resources to enforce the law. Nevertheless, word got around in a small place and it wouldn't have been worth Robert's father's reputation to have even a sniff of an ale wife's apron in one of Kirkintilloch's drop houses.

This afternoon, there was more than a touch of the disreputable about the Anchor and the wife serving behind the bar. She was amiable enough though, and the few patrons dotted about the premises, while not welcoming, were not overtly hostile either.

Robert stood at the bar and asked for a whisky. The alewife motioned to him with an outstretched hand, and he rummaged in his pocket for some coins. The paucity of those he retrieved were testament to the others he had squandered on getting rid of his harasser near the Green. He paid for his drink before she served it. When it arrived, he took a sip and suppressed a grimace as the liquid scalded his throat.

'Thank you,' he said, coughing despite his best efforts to appear accustomed to so coarse a strain of alcohol. He nodded in the direction of the barmaid, who acknowledged him before hoisting herself onto a tall, three-legged stool and leaning back against the wall, surveying her domain. Her clothes were drab and dirty looking, but the plaid shawl draped over her shoulders was secured by an amber coloured brooch that was highly polished and gleamed when it caught the light of a candle burning in a sconce above the rows of bottles and tumblers. She had a fine head of thick, dark hair but her face was wrinkled and pock-marked and her mouth so downturned that Robert couldn't imagine an event joyous enough to provoke even the smallest flicker of a smile from it. She looked middle-aged at the very least, but he knew she was probably under thirty.

He sipped his whisky tentatively and perused the barroom and its patrons from his vantage point. The room consisted of a narrow rectangle with the bar running along most of the length of one wall. A door at the end of it looked like it led to a back room or a large storage press. A variety of seating was arranged opposite the bar; old wooden tables and a collection of mismatched stools for the most part, a settle on each side of the fire and a couple of benches like church pews, which were shoved into a recess to make a kind of rudimentary anteroom. The only light was afforded by two small windows set into the upper portion of wall facing the street, a single candle burning in the sconce, and the occasional shaft of daylight that crept in through the K-shape of the hooked curtain at the Anchor's entrance.

A group of four older men were sitting at a table directly across from him, playing cards. They all had the care-worn aspect he had come to expect of the labouring class, heavyset frames with muscles turning slowly to fat, a taciturn aspect to each of their faces. Robert watched as one of the men folded his cards onto the table with a sigh and some money exchanged hands. They all wore the same rough uniform of open necked shirt and belted drab breeches, garments rarely washed and never ironed.

They were the kind of people whose bodies seemed to have been sapped of all the stores of energy that God had originally gifted them. Gruelling physical work had built them up so brutally that, when they became too old to hew into the earth or shoulder weighted burdens for hours on end, they simply depleted. Like a bellows, which, having taken in as much air as it could hold, shrank and sagged once it had done its job. There would be no easy retirement for any of these men, Robert thought. They would be expected to scrape some kind of living into their old age and, if they were lucky, die quickly and efficiently in a son or daughter's crowded room rather than suffer the protracted humiliation of parish relief. He thought of his own father, gravely ill these past five years, his chest constricted as a result of the inhalation of flax fibres over his lifetime. And yet, he lingered on, not unhappily, tended by his family, safe in the knowledge that they would look after him until he departed the world and ensure he was buried, and his resting place marked by a stone.

At home, as long as the weather was dry, he and

Maggie would take the pupils out on Saturdays. He often took the older boys for a climb up Salisbury Crags while Maggie and Isabella took the girls and the younger children around Duddingston Loch, to run and play and feed the ducks and swans. Physical activity that contributed to the children's health and wellbeing, the contact with nature both pleasurable and uplifting. The world and his experiences in it had improved because he had been lucky. Lucky to grow up in a stable family, lucky to have had an education thanks to the generous support and encouragement of Mr and Mrs Watt in Kirkintilloch and his parents' willingness to allow him to forego the flax-dressing trade.

Robert took another sip of the whisky. It didn't taste as bad now that he had got a little used to it.

Two young men were having an argument at the far end of the bar. What had started off as whispered insults and asides had developed into a bit of a shouting match and Robert worried that it might build into a full-blown fight. They seemed to be talking about a woman and, from the snippets he had overheard so far, Robert suspected the first lad was being accused of letting down or committing some kind of outrage on the second lad's sister. The accused was tall and solid-looking, the second man, smaller and slighter, was almost on his tiptoes, squaring up to his adversary. All of sudden, though, an older man that Robert had not seen ambled out of the shadows and cuffed the second lad across the top of the head, knocking him near off his feet. The first lad laughed like a drain at this turn of events, while the second seemed bewildered, so consumed with frustration and aggression had he been that he seemed to still be piecing together what had actually happened. Then the older man laughed and put his arm around the boy he had just assailed. Within a few seconds all three of them were amiable again, proposing toasts with a new round of drinks, the previous issue forgotten.

The alewife approached Robert, bottle in hand.

'Do you want another?'

'No thank you. I'm fine for now,' Robert said.

'Keeping a clear heid, are you?'

'Trying to. I'm here on an errand.'

She surveyed him with a look that he thought suggested circumspection as opposed to outright suspicion, so Robert decided to carry on with his enquiry.

'I'm looking for a man by the name of James Donnelly. I believe he lives near here?'

She surveyed him in silence for a few moments.

Robert pressed on. 'I've been commissioned to help defend a deaf woman called Jean Campbell. She's currently in the Edinburgh Tolbooth charged with the murder of an infant.'

'Oh, aye. I know Jean Campbell. You won't find many around here that don't know of the case.'

Another silence ensued while the alewife continued to size him up and Robert tried not to look uncomfortable.

We'll be here all day, he thought. Robert decided to take the initiative.

'My name's Kinniburgh, I'm a teacher at the Deaf and Dumb Institution in Edinburgh. I'm trying to understand what happened to Jean so that I can help her. She's very reluctant to talk to the authorities.'

The alewife looked at him with suspicion.

Robert hoisted his bag onto the bar and pulled out one of his pamphlets. He flattened it and laid it out between them, pointing to the illustration of the institution on the front.

'I can communicate by signs with deaf people. I'm trying to do that with Jean. I think she may have been badly treated. She swears she did not murder her child. I'm trying to find out what really happened.'

At this, the ale wife's affected disinterest fell away.

'Of course she didn't kill her child! I don't know much. I might not be able to read they words on your bit of paper, but I do know that she never killed that wean. Lassie didnae have it in her to harm a child.'

'I see, Mrs . . .? Excuse me, I don't know your name.'

'Helen Shannon, but most folk just call me Nell.'

'Nell, I would be most grateful if you would tell me what you know of this unfortunate woman. I am finding it difficult to understand some of her story. Partly because she is reluctant to divulge certain facts – perhaps they are too painful – but also because I understand little of what her life was like in the months leading up to her arrest.'

Nell dragged her stool along the floor and set it opposite Robert.

'Are you telling me the truth, Mr Kinniburgh? I wouldnae be saying anything that might hurt Jean?'

'No,' Robert said, 'whatever you say can only assist me. I have Jean's best interests at heart.'

Nell nodded.

'And she's alright, the lassie? In that prison, I mean.'

'She's safe,' said Robert. 'You should have no worries in that respect. It is a basic place, and no one would want to be divested of their liberty, but I have seen her, and she is as comfortable as can be expected, under the circumstances.'

Nell's eyes watered. 'It's a long way away. Edinburgh, I mean. It's not what she's used to.'

Robert looked at her, incredulously. 'It's not so far. Or so different from Glasgow, for that matter. I came from there by coach myself only yesterday.'

'Indeed? I've never been out of Glasgow in my life, sir. I can't imagine having the means to go as far as the capital.'

'But your name – Shannon – is Irish,' said Robert. 'Surely you travelled from that country? Or were you born here of Irish parents?'

Nell shook her head. 'I was only married to an Irishman, Mr Kinniburgh, and he's long gone.'

'I am sorry for your loss,' Robert said.

'Oh, he didn't die. He just left one day and never came back. Right enough, I don't know for definite that he's alive either. No real loss though. You'll think this a terrible thing to say, sir, but I'm much better off without him. He was a terrible man for wasting hard-earned money. The Anchor might be rough but it's a decent living.'

'Jean tells me that the man she lived with, Jim, is an Irishman. Is that right?'

'He is,' said Nell. 'From Donegal, originally, like my absent husband. Although my man came from Aran Island and Donnelly from Dungloe, I believe. He's a passable enough fellow. Handy with his fists from time to time but most of them around this place are. A lot of them feel they have to act the hard man if they want left alone.'

'And he and Jean, how did they get along together?' Robert asked.

Nell laughed. 'Well, she was something different to what we were used to. The lassie couldnae hear a thing and she'd came from a decent family in the Calton.'

One of the two young men at the end of the bar banged on the counter for service and Nell turned towards him. She shot him a look that implied he would get no service if he carried on in that vein and he held up his hand in a drunken apology. She waited for a beat, just to make sure he was aware that she was at no man's beck and call, and then moved to serve him.

In a few moments she was back.

'Where might I find this man Donnelly?' Robert asked.

'He has lodgings in Taylor's Close,' Nell said. 'If you go out of here and turn right, then right again, you'll find yourself on the Briggait. Walk along a wee bit and the entrance to the close is directly opposite the Merchants' Hall. I don't know if Jim'll be there, mind.'

Robert thanked Nell. He used most of the money he had left on him to give her a decent tip and she curled the coins in her palm, casting her eyes around the room to check if anyone had noticed. Satisfied, she tucked the money inside a leather pouch around her waist and tied it securely.

24

~ Tuesday, 4 March 1817:
Taylor's Close, Glasgow ~

Robert was surprised to find that the area around the Saltmarket and Briggait reminded him of much of Edinburgh. Higgledy-piggledy houses and hastily thrown-up businesses with corbie-stepped cables and tiled roofs. Impossibly narrow vennels leading to dark, dank closes where humankind jostled for position and did their best to survive in unsanitary conditions. As he crossed King Street, the stench of dead animal was quite overpowering; mutton mixed with beef mixed with fish. Like an enormous stew baking in the marketplace. Carts clattered past, some piled high with animal carcasses and sacks of newly caught fish heading to the markets and some with boxed joints of lamb and beef, herring and haddock being rushed back out of the centre to shops in adjoining towns and villages or towards the river to be loaded and shipped out of the city to some far-flung trading post.

Robert spotted the Merchants' Hall on the south side of the road. It was an impressive structure, a two-storey building with a huge steeple, at least 150 feet high, with a copper ship on a globe in place of a weathervane. The structure had a pleasing symmetry, with elegant pediments to the upper row of windows. There were a couple of shops open on the ground floor and an arched entranceway in the middle. A large brass clock took up a section in the middle of the tower and Robert noticed the time; almost half past three.

The sky had turned ominously cloudy, and Robert hurried on, keen to complete his errand before the rain started. He crossed the road and cut down the nearest vennel. There was no indication of the street name but a wooden sign reading 'Chas. Taylor, Grocer' gave him some confidence he had chosen the right path.

A young woman, knee deep in small children, was in conversation with another woman who was leaning out of a ground-floor window, her bare arms resting on the grimy sill. Both women had their sleeves pushed up beyond their elbows, their skin raw-looking, as if it had been flayed like the beasts in the markets. Robert, emboldened, approached them.

'Is this Taylor's Close?' he asked.

The woman who was standing nodded while the one who was inside the house gestured towards an area where the cramped pathway seemed to open out. 'Aye. It's Taylor's right up to that gable end.'

'I'm looking for a fellow by the name of Donnelly. Would you know where I might enquire after him?'

'Aye,' said the second woman, from the frame of her window, 'see where that cart's rested? If you go through the doorway there, he's in one of the rooms off the main stairwell. Might be the second floor he stays on?' She looked at her companion for clarification, but the other woman just shrugged.

Robert thanked them.

He walked gingerly along the vennel, taking care on cobbles that were slick with greasy water in places. Old, peeling bill posters were dotted here and there, advertising household products, long-past hiring fair days and penny geggies on the Green. A tall tenement stretched up on his right-hand side, to the left were a series of older, smaller buildings, some still with thatched roofs. Washing poles sprouted from underneath windows, a pair of large men's trousers hung limp in the stale air, like a weary flag. The smell here was of ash mounds and middens.

At the end of the vennel was a wider court where a group of boys sat talking and smoking. They stared blankly at Robert as he crossed to the entrance next to the cart. There was no door as such, but a metal surround had been erected, like a tall, shallow porch. The metal was patterned with a grille at the top. It looked like it had been repurposed rather than being a bespoke addition to the house. The threshold acted as a bridge across an open sewer that ran the length of the wall. The soles of Robert's shoes clanged as he stepped upon it.

A tortoiseshell cat, which had been lurking at the foot of the stairs, emerged and wound itself around Robert's ankles, meowing. Riddled with fleas, he thought. Despite his better judgement, he leant down to scritch its head and the cat pushed its cheek to his palm, flicking its head to persuade Robert to stroke it. He hunkered down and looked into its yellow eyes.

'I've got nothing for you, wee cat.'

Robert stood up and went up the first flight of stairs. The cat followed him. He knocked at the first door he came to but there was no answer. However, the door across the landing opened and a young girl, no older than six or seven, peered out.

'Hello,' he said, 'do you know where Mr Donnelly stays?'

'In that one,' the girl replied, pointing to the door Robert had already tried. 'He's no there the day, but.'

'Do you know when he'll be back?'

She shook her head. 'He's gone away, mister. With a gang of men for to work on the canal. My da's gone with them.'

'Do you know when they'll be back?'

She shook her head again. 'My ma might. She's inside.'

Robert smiled at the girl. 'Could you ask her for me?'

After a couple of moments, a woman appeared, her head tilted to one side, appraising this unexpected caller. She wiped her hands on her apron and rested them on her hips.

'You looking for Jim?' she said.

'Yes,' said Robert, 'it's about his . . . about Jean Campbell. Your daughter told me he's away working. Do you have any idea when he'll be back?'

'The whole job was to last ten days, my man's due back sometime on Saturday or Sunday.'

Robert was disappointed. He had hoped to see Jim Donnelly as soon as possible.

'I'm no sure if all the men are away till then. A fair few dinnae bide the night. It depends how far away they're put to work.'

'Can I leave you my name? If Mr Donnelly should return this evening, I'd be very grateful if you would ask him to come to see me. I shall make it worth his while. I'm at the Tontine Hotel. If he asks for Mr Kinniburgh, I'll make sure they know to pass his message on.'

Robert rummaged in his pocket and brought out a card of introduction from the institution. He pointed at his name.

'This is me,' he said.

'At the Tontine, you say?'

Robert nodded.

The woman took the card from him and put it in the pocket of her apron. She made to close the door and Robert said, quickly, 'Please make sure he knows I mean him well.'

25

~ *Tuesday, 4 March 1817:*
Calton, Glasgow ~

Angus was holding forth on the plight of his parishioners. He was preaching to the converted, as his audience consisted of his son and the teacher of the capital's Deaf and Dumb Institution, but the minister carried on regardless.

It is unfortunate that the deaf are not treated in the same way as the hearing. The idea that lack of hearing or speech is connected with intelligence is widespread and it holds people back.

Robert was hungrily tucking into his dinner. He had returned to the Calton after completing his enquiries as to Jim Donnelly's whereabouts. He wasn't used to drinking in the afternoon, and the questionable spirits he had imbibed in the Anchor had given him a headache, but the mutton stew and freshly baked bannocks that Mrs Buchanan had put in front of him were having a restorative effect.

Angus gestured to David.

During my own son's childhood, I could see no prospect for him. There was nowhere he could go to receive an education. I decided to teach him myself. Later, when I saw that he suffered from lack of contact with children his own age and with those who were also deaf, I began to make connections with other deaf people and started the church as a way for them to worship and find like-minded society. The education I was able to furnish David with is no doubt much inferior to that of your school in Edinburgh, but I like to think he has done well for himself, despite having been born with what people view as such a disadvantage.

Robert put down his knife and fork. *I'm sure he's a credit to you,* he signed.

David took up the story.

I am now apprenticed to a jeweller. I can read and write thanks to the efforts of my father, but I can also make signs and be understood by other deaf people. It is important that we can all be a support to one another.

And what of the younger deaf? Robert asked. *Are you able to help them?*

David nodded. *The church, and my father's work, started to be more widely known in Glasgow and the surrounding areas. People know what we are doing here and contact my father to find out if we can help their children. We have a Sunday school now. My mother and I run it while my father conducts the main service. Unfortunately, only those who live nearby are able to come.*

It is difficult to educate children who are scattered far and wide, Robert replied. *In my own school, the richer families pay for tuition and accommodation, but we have been lucky to attract some generous benefactors who fund places for poorer children. Deafness is no respecter of social circumstances.*

We will improve things, won't we? Angus said. *With God's will and the help of the good people of Glasgow, perhaps we will be able to set up a similar institution to your own, Robert. Or, at the very least, provide the means to send children to be educated by your good self.*

Mrs Buchanan appeared with a dish of treacle sponge and some bowls. She sat down to join the men as they all helped themselves to a piece.

Angus cleared his throat. 'I hope you don't mind, Robert, but we were hoping you might return in your capacity as teacher when time allows? When news of your present visit reached me, some of our committee asked to meet you. They're very eager to hear of your progress in Edinburgh.'

Robert caught David's eye and answered in signs.

I would be happy to talk to them. Will the deaf be invited too?

I don't see why not, said Angus. *If they wish.*

Everyone agreed that they would be very interested to hear what Robert had to say and David asked, *Will it be done using signs?*

Yes. Of course, said Robert. *I will sign to the deaf and speak to the hearing. There is no point, to my mind, discussing the wellbeing of deaf people unless they are able to understand what I'm saying. I'd like to demonstrate my methods as I've done at previous meetings, but I have no pupils in Glasgow with whom to do so.* He glanced at David. *Would you be willing to help me?*

David smiled. *I would be happy to.*

'Who would you expect to come along?' Robert asked Angus.

'The gentlemen of the city who make up our small committee. From the Trades' Hall and the Merchants' Hall. They are reputable men who have climbed the ranks of their respective professions. They wish to contribute to the general good and are interested in helping me fund these endeavours. I am sure they will be only too happy to spread the word and encourage their colleagues to reach into their pockets.'

26

~ Tuesday, 4 March 1817:
The Tontine Hotel, Glasgow ~

Robert was more than ready for his bed, but he ordered a drink at the bar and lingered there a while, draping his greatcoat on a stool and setting down his bag at his feet.

A small number of residents and visitors still peppered the seats, smoking pipes and sipping quietly at glasses of spirits and cups of coffee and hot chocolate. A huge grandfather clock stood in a corner of the room, its rhythm counting down to the end of the day. Some glasses were set out on a draining board and when the barman used his apron to dry them, the linen squeaked as he pushed it into the damp corners. Robert watched as a moth fluttered around a branch of the ornate candelabra that burned beside him on the bar counter.

He had one or two mouthfuls of whisky and then decided to take his glass to his room. He didn't particularly wish to be alone but neither did he want to drink in a room full of strangers. More than anything, he wanted to talk to his wife, to have the opportunity to discuss and dissect his day with someone who understood his work and shared his view of the world. Margaret would need no preamble, would not require too much context or explanation. He would write a letter to Succoth and enclose it within another to Margaret. He would give an account of the day just passed and outline his plans for the next.

He could ask Margaret to deliver Succoth's letter. If the letters went on the overnight coach, they would arrive in Edinburgh by the next morning.

Upstairs, he took up pen and paper and settled himself at the small desk in the corner of his room. Outside the window the sky was pitch-black, but the city still thrummed with noise and street lamps continued to burn. He went into his case and took out a scroll of battered leather, tied in the middle. He unwrapped it and got out a few sheets of paper and some of his writing implements. He used a cloth to wipe off some dust that had gathered on the nib of his pen, unscrewed a pot of Indian ink, dipped his pen and began to write.

27

~ *Wednesday, 5 March 1817:*
Briggait, Glasgow ~

Robert breakfasted late and, afterwards, took himself a hundred yards or so along the Trongate. Using more of Lord Succoth's allowance, he booked his seat on a stage-coach leaving the following day.

By mid-morning, he was in the police office at the Bridge-end. He sat on a bench that ran the length of the wall. Opposite was an imposing counter over which a rangy desk sergeant held sway. Robert had approached him around ten minutes previously and announced that he was there to speak to Sergeant McLeod; the police officer who had been on duty at the time of Jean's arrest.

The police office was already lively, and the desk sergeant waved Robert away to wait on the convenience of McLeod, who was believed to be somewhere in the station and who would be sent for just as soon as was practicable. A group of three constables were standing at the desk, each holding fast to the folk they had recently apprehended, waiting to deliver their collars into the custody of the sergeant behind the desk.

Robert was glad that the police had uniforms, otherwise, he mused, he might have found it difficult to distinguish the upholders of the law from those who had broken it. All of the policemen he had seen so far had scars and bruises of one kind or another that were remarkably similar to those of their charges.

Next to him on the bench was a young girl whose nose and upper lip were covered in dried blood, and a very frail, elderly man who seemed to have come into the station primarily for a sit down and a heat beside the fireplace.

Eventually, the desk sergeant beckoned Robert back to the tall counter and sent him off along a corridor, where he was met by McLeod, a tall man with ruddy cheeks and short, spiky dark hair. He had rather pointed eyebrows that lent him an air of permanent surprise.

'Hallo, Mr Kinniburgh, please come straight through,' McLeod said, in an accent that marked him as being of Highland descent. 'You'll be wanting to know about the Campbell woman's case?'

'Yes, I've read your report, Sergeant McLeod, so I know the bare bones of the case, but I'm particularly interested in what your impression was of Jean when you arrested her.'

'Well,' McLeod began, 'there was a right stramash going on by the time I got to the bridge. A lot of shouting and pushing from the crowd that had gathered. My immediate task was to hold those people back, identify any witnesses and get the woman safely into the police office before she came to any harm.'

'Were you aware that she was deaf when you apprehended her?'

'Not at first,' said McLeod. 'To be honest, I didn't really pay her much attention until I got her inside and, even then, it took some more time to establish that she couldn't hear rather than wouldn't speak. The crowd had been shouting about her throwing a child off the bridge but, at that stage, I wasn't sure if she had done it deliberately or if it had been an accident. In fact, in the absence of a body, I wasn't completely sure it had happened at all. It was only after we identified the two witnesses that I began to get a clearer picture. And, by that time, the chances of locating the poor child's body had decreased considerably.'

Robert nodded. 'Indeed. I believe the boatman has had no luck in finding it?'

'Not for the want of trying on his part,' said McLeod. 'But it had been raining heavily for days before the incident and the river was fast-flowing. The boatman thinks it likely that the child was swept westward almost instantly.'

'So, the body could have ended up miles away within hours?' Robert asked.

'Exactly so. The Humane Society do good work and they've retrieved people both dead and alive in all weathers, but the Clyde is a busy river and full of detritus from the city. It's not the easiest place to search for a body that small. Even if the weather conditions hadn't been against him, there's no guarantee that the boatman could have retrieved it.'

'I see,' said Robert. 'And Jean Campbell, I know you couldn't communicate with her but how did she seem when you brought her back here? Was she obviously distressed? The witness statements suggest she appeared unsteady on her feet and that she might have been drunk, but she denies that.'

'I don't think she was drunk, Mr Kinniburgh,' said McLeod. 'She was shaky, and she looked like she'd been in a fight very recently. She had a cut above her eye and over the few hours we had her in custody here, there were fresh bruises visible on her arms and around her neck.'

'Did a doctor examine her?'

McLeod shook his head.

'Why not?'

'Mr Kinniburgh, if we paid a doctor to examine every-body who comes through these doors with cuts and bruises, the city would be bankrupt in a week. I suppose if we'd known this would turn out to be a murder case, we might have looked more closely at Jean Campbell's injuries but, as it was, she looked like just another woman who had taken a beating, either from a stranger or her own man.'

'I realise this is just conjecture on your part, Mr McLeod, but do you think the bruising around her neck is significant? Might someone have tried to strangle her?'

McLeod gave this a moment's thought.

'It's possible. Although there's women in the streets around here get a doing from their men daily and just accept it as a matter of course. They've no choice but to put up with it.'

'And the law can't intervene?' Robert asked.

McLeod laughed mirthlessly. 'There would be no room in the cells for the real criminals if we did. Violence is a way of life for these folk and how a man treats his wife in his own home is his own business.'

'Jean Campbell's injuries wouldn't have seemed significant?'

'No, Mr Kinniburgh, that they would not.'

~

Robert stood for some considerable time on the Old Bridge. The Trongate's distant bell marked the hour as five o'clock in the evening. Glasgow was already shrouded in darkness, and chill winds lurked in every alley. On the face of it, conditions were similar to those of almost two weeks since.

He tried to imagine what had happened that night. Bruised and battered, Jean had stood in the middle of a bridge on a busy thoroughfare in the largest city in Scotland, but she would barely have been visible. The few lamps cast only a small amount of light. The evening, then as now, was dull and overcast.

133

According to the two young men who had given statements to the police, Jean had staggered slightly, giving the
impression that she was the worse for drink, while people
around her hurried to their next destination, reluctant to
linger. The area around the Briggait had been flooded with
immigrants in recent years – particularly those from Ireland.
Glasgow imagined itself a modern, vibrant city but its
poorer inhabitants were subject to the vagaries of industry
and commerce. On the bridge, Jean's dress and demeanour
would have marked her out as undesirable at best and
dispensable at worst.

Robert found it easy to conjure a picture of Jean standing
beside him. Her head and face shrouded by a shawl, her
shapeless gown and heavy boots making her slight frame
appear bulkier than was, in fact, the case. She would have
clutched the bundle she was carrying to her chest and leant
on the wooden bridge to steady herself.

The bundle had spilled onto the parapet of the bridge.
Robert imagined it rolling forward and Jean lunging at it,
trying to grab it back but, although the tips of her fingers
might have reached it, she wasn't quick enough, and the
bundle continued to fall, greeting the Clyde with a splash
and sinking so quickly into the inky black water that it was
almost as if it had never existed.

A sharp, high-pitched cry had rung out briefly and
floated into the night. Jean would have turned and hurried
along the pavement in the direction of the tollhouse on the
Gorbals side of the river.

Now, the scant attention that passers-by paid her had
become, unexpectedly, valuable. These fragments had been
knitted together; destined to make up something resembling
the truth.

28

∼ Wednesday, 5 March 1817:
Chessels Court, Edinburgh ∼

Margaret unfolded her letter and re-read it. She had rushed to the Post Office that evening, to find out if anything had arrived on the stage from Glasgow. Sure enough, there were two letters awaiting collection. One, Robert's letter to Succoth, was to be dropped off at His Lordship's chambers, and the other, which she now held in her hands, was for her alone.

At first, she was fair taken with its receipt. It had been dark when she journeyed to the High Street to collect it. She had hurried back to the school and gone directly upstairs for some peace and quiet. She should have been helping Isabella to clear up the supper things, but she wasn't prepared to wait until that was done to find out what Robert had to say. He had only been gone two nights, but his absence was such an unusual thing and a letter from her husband was a novelty in itself, regardless of its contents.

As it transpired, Robert's letter was a little underwhelming. It performed all the functions that a satisfactory letter should, but it did not fulfil Margaret's hopes and expectations. Robert's tone was disappointingly even and his expressions of emotion slightly too muted for Margaret's liking. But then, what had she been expecting? An upstanding schoolteacher such as Robert was unlikely to disclose his deepest, darkest longings in print, even to his wife. Nevertheless, he owned that he missed her. Perhaps that was enough, thought Margaret, as she folded the letter and tucked it in a drawer in her bedside cabinet.

29

~ Thursday, 6 March 1817:
The Tontine Hotel, Glasgow ~

Robert went downstairs and settled his bill. One of the lads from the hotel took his case and strapped it onto the top railings of the coach that stood, uncoupled from its horses, on the north side of Argyle Street.

It had rained heavily overnight, and the pock-marked street was a mass of dirty puddles. The rising sun burned through what clouds remained, beckoning in what promised to be a fine morning. Robert perched on a tall stool at a broad windowsill that looked out onto the busy thoroughfare. He was leafing through one of the newspapers placed there for the convenience of the Tontine's patrons, but his eye was drawn outside, where all manner of people bustled by.

A group of urchins, barefoot in the opening to a close on the opposite side of the street, caught his eye. Three little boys, playing with a ball made of scraps and bound with rags. They kicked it along the narrow alleyway, and it bounced in the filthy puddles that had collected in a loose patchwork of paving stones. The three boys disappeared into the gloomy close mouth but one of them must have taken an almighty kick at the ball, because a moment later, it came shooting out into the path of a labourer who was carrying some tools along the street. The startled man tripped and stumbled in such a comical fashion that the boy who ran out to retrieve the ball began to laugh. The furious labourer, having righted himself, struck the lad so hard on the back of his head that his laughter turned to tears and the chastened child retreated into the safety of the alleyway.

Robert considered ordering another coffee and then thought better of it. The coach would be leaving shortly, and he didn't much fancy being jolted all the way to their first stop with a full bladder. Sure enough, he spotted four horses being led out from the mews at the back of the Tontine by a couple of stable hands. He watched as the lads coupled the beasts to their harnesses and lined each pair up. The horses whinnied and stamped but were soon mollified into submission.

The Tontine's doorman, the buttons of his waistcoat straining to contain his stomach, called through from his spot at the entrance to the hotel.

'Passengers for the Edinburgh stage!'

Robert slid down from the stool, put on his hat and picked up his brown leather bag. He wrapped his green muffler around his neck and traipsed outside, along with a middle-aged couple who had been sitting at a table nearby.

Outside, the sun was getting stronger, but a chill wind prevailed and wound itself around the small group of people who congregated at the side of the coach. As well as Robert and the couple who had followed him outside, there were two other passengers – two young men who Robert took to be brothers. Both had the same distinctive close-set eyes, the colour of bluebells.

Inside the coach, Robert sat alongside the brothers, letting the couple have more room to themselves on the opposite bench. The seats on this coach were better upholstered than the ones on his journey through to Glasgow and once they set off, the motion of the carriage on the well-surfaced road out of the city lulled Robert into a slumber.

When the postillion blew his horn from outside the

carriage, Robert woke with a start and no idea of how long they had been travelling. In a few minutes, however, they pulled into a small inn that occupied an exposed position in the midst of moorland. It was called the Mitre, but the name gave Robert no clue as to its location. The innkeeper and stable hand, alerted by the noise of the horn, had come out to receive their visitors.

He asked the husband of the couple if he knew where they were.

'Just outside Camelon, I believe,' the man replied, continuing when he saw Robert's confused expression. 'Near Falkirk. If you look down the glen, you can make out a stretch of the canal.'

Robert peered out the dirty window and could spy a straight line of blue in the distance.

~

Within the Mitre, Robert ordered a large pot of coffee and offered to share it with his fellow passengers.

Mr and Mrs Bolter were travelling back to their home in Edinburgh, having combined a business trip with visits to friends in Glasgow. Mr Bolter supplied machinery for excavation and was involved, in a minor way, with both the works to clear the Nor Loch and the proposed new canal that would transport coal and other goods from Falkirk to Edinburgh.

The elder of the young men, Michael McGroarty, was accompanying his younger brother, Daniel, who was due to take up a place with a new brewery that had been established in the city. The lad's new workplace, it transpired, was at Fountainbridge, next to a canal basin that Bolter was working on. The group of passengers sat companionably for half an hour or so, until the horses had been fed and watered and the coachmen called to them to embark once again. Robert was friendly and solicitous but vague about the reasons for his own journey. He mentioned that he was a teacher at the Deaf and Dumb Institution and there were murmurs of approval at this and questions as to the nature of sign language. Robert took pains not to mention the Jean Campbell case and, instead, steered the conversation to the new pleasure gardens intended for the site of the drained Nor Loch.

~

The night was clear and remarkably clement by the time they reached Edinburgh. A crescent moon hung white against a navy-blue sky and Robert stretched out his limbs and studied the constellations as he waited for his bags to be unloaded from the stage.

The High Street was all but deserted as the small knot of passengers said their goodbyes, each of them wishing the young McGroarty luck in his new job. A carter was positioned near the steps of the Post Office and Mr Bolter hailed him.

'We live near the Pleasance,' said Mrs Bolter. 'Are you headed in that direction? You'd be welcome to put your bags on the cart.'

'Thank you. I'll go the length of the Canongate, Mrs Bolter, but you must let me contribute to the cost.' Robert fumbled in his jacket for his pocketbook.

Mrs Bolter shook her head. 'Put your money away. It's all one to us and we'd appreciate your company at this late hour. You never know who you might meet in one of these dark alleyways!'

The carter heaved their trunks onto his vehicle and Robert added his bags to the pile.

'You'll be glad to get home, Mr Kinniburgh,' Mrs Bolter said, as they approached Chessels Court. 'There's nothing like your own bed to sleep in.'

'I will that,' Robert agreed.

'I'm sure your wife and children will be happy to have you back from your travels.'

'My wife and I haven't been blessed with children as yet,' said Robert.

'I'm sure it's only a matter of time, Mr Kinniburgh, until you've bairns under your feet,' Mrs Bolter said, smiling as she bid him farewell.

The house was in darkness when he arrived home and Margaret sleeping. Robert took off his greatcoat and left his baggage in the hallway so as not to disturb her. His unpacking could be done in the morning. He was dog-tired and his own bed was as tempting as Mrs Bolter had predicted.

30

∼ Friday, 10 January 1817:
Partickhill Road, Glasgow ∼

Euphemia sat at the bureau in the small upstairs sitting room and leafed through the pages of the *Scots Magazine*. The New Year's edition was satisfyingly crammed with domestic and international news as well as sundry ephemera and advertisements. Euphemia was quite capable of devouring the whole publication in one sitting but, as ever, she endeavoured to make it last by limiting herself to a few pages each day.

This morning, she was engrossed in an article about an abortive mission to the Congo to find the source of the Niger. In the early days of their union, she might have slipped a bookmark between these pages and attempted to discuss it with her husband over dinner. She would have supposed him interested in a project that utilised cargo ships and barges to discover hitherto untamed lands. However, Charles had not turned out to be a man of intellect, or even basic curiosity.

Euphemia's concentration faltered as a series of thumps and scrapes from the far end of the hallway pressed in on her consciousness. Martha had been tasked with turning out the nursery in preparation for the deaf woman's arrival the following day. Euphemia picked at a ragged edge of skin on her bottom lip and winced as it ripped. Charles's baby manufactory was being conjured into life and there was nothing that she could do to stop it.

∼

In the nursery, Martha was on her hands and knees scrubbing the wooden floor. The sweep had been called in the week before and Martha had already polished the mantelpiece and washed down the furniture in readiness for the deaf mother and her unborn baby. Now, the window was pushed open, and she was busy cleaning every corner of the room. Tomorrow she would make up the bed and bassinet with clean linen.

A sharp wind blew in and Martha got up to close the window. She wondered what this new stranger would make of the view of grassland and meadow that stretched out to the west, the Hay Burn winding between groups of trees. Would she think it a fine aspect or would its emptiness make her feel lonely and miss her home in the city?

Martha felt almost giddy with excitement at the prospect of these new additions to the household. At first, when Ina had explained how the master and mistress were adopting a poor deaf and dumb woman's baby, she had been surprised and anxious. Once Ina had explained that it would be a kindness both for the poor mother herself and the mistress, who would be spared the toll of further pregnancies, Martha had grown accustomed to the idea. She had never met a deaf person before. The master had said that this woman communicated by signs and they would all be able to converse with her with a little practice.

∼

Downstairs, Charles was similarly disturbed by Martha's readying of the nursery. He had intended to spend the forenoon catching up on his business correspondence, but the anticipation of the Campbell woman's arrival seemed to encroach on his every effort. Now, he could neither sit at peace nor find any occupation that would curb his anxiety.

143

He drained the dregs of his tea and poured into the cup a small amount of malt whisky from a decanter on the sideboard. The amber fluid swirled with black flecks of tealeaves and he knocked the mixture back in one. He wasn't generally given to drinking before midday, but he felt the need for a straightener. Not that he was in any doubt as to the advisability of this course of action. It was a necessary step. His wife might have her uses as a conduit to the Rintoul coffers but as a source of offspring she was wholly unreliable.

Charles helped himself to another measure and drank it in two gulps this time. The warm liquid functioned as a balm to his unease. There was nothing to worry over. They were doing this woman a kindness, and she, them. The money that would be exchanged was simply a by-product of their charity. All would be well. He would have an heir to secure Rintoul's adherence, Euphemia would be relieved of her child-bearing responsibilities, and Jean Campbell would safeguard her child's future.

31

∼ Friday, 7 March 1817:
The Tolbooth Prison, Edinburgh ∼

The door to Jean's cell was ajar. Inside, Robert was taken aback to find a smartly dressed man of about sixty years, and a surgeon's bag atop the deal table. He was further discomfited to discover that Jean herself was not present.

He cleared his throat. 'I'm looking for the prisoner, Jean Campbell.'

The man stood up and proffered a hand. He was small, of a compact build. His clothes, though crumpled and worn, were made of the best material. He had a thick mop of white hair and untamed whiskers that threatened to overwhelm his face.

'You'll be Kinniburgh, no doubt? I'm Dr Edwin Browne. I'm here at Lord Succoth's request. His Lordship told me you'd likely be in attendance today.'

The two men shook hands.

'Pleased to meet you, doctor,' said Robert. 'Is Jean poorly?'

'Not at all,' Browne assured him. 'In point of fact, she's in remarkably good health, given the circumstances. I was sent by His Lordship to examine her. Medically, that is. I've no intention of stepping on your toes.'

'I didn't realise a physical examination was necessary,' said Robert.

'It isn't as a rule,' explained Dr Browne. 'A medical is only ordered if there is any doubt as to whether the panel is able to undergo a trial. If there is a suggestion that a prisoner is physically or mentally unfit, Succoth can move to have them committed to a hospital or an asylum rather than mount a prosecution.'

'Why would His Lordship want to do that?' Robert asked, 'I thought he was keen to see justice done?'

Dr Browne shrugged, 'It costs a lot to take a case to trial and this is no ordinary case. I wouldn't presume to know the mind of Lord Succoth, but he'll want to make sure there's no alternative before he spends the crown's money.'

'He can't just shut people away, though?' Robert argued. 'Everyone has a right to a fair trial.'

Dr Browne gave a dry laugh. 'You'd be surprised at how many inconvenient defendants find their way into our institutions, Mr Kinniburgh. Nevertheless, if Succoth wants Jean Campbell out of the way, I'll not be the man that signs the papers.'

'You don't think there's anything wrong with her?'

Dr Browne shook his head. 'She's deaf, alright, but as far as I can see she has no indication of mental deficiencies or lunacy or any physical health problem, other than the usual lice and such.'

'And where is she now, doctor?'

'Along the corridor getting dressed,' Dr Browne said. 'Before I examined her, I got her to have a bath. You never know what state prisoners will be in, although Mr Sibbald runs a tight ship here, depleted as it is at the moment.'

'Lord Succoth won't be happy then?' Robert asked.

The doctor shrugged again. 'I wouldn't know. He may well be delighted that he can go ahead with the trial. I'm a medical man, Mr Kinniburgh, what I know about the intricacies of the legal system could be carved on the head of a pin.'

There was a clattering sound from another part of the prison and Dr Browne winked.

'Mr Sibbald, on the other hand, is definitely not happy. He's had to fetch and carry water from the basement up three flights of stairs and, if I'm not mistaken, is now struggling to get the tin bath back down again.'

Robert smiled. He was warming to Dr Browne. The medical man's tone, which had, at first, seemed perfunctory, he now suspected was merely pragmatic.

'Which hospital are you employed at, Dr Browne?' asked Robert.

'The Royal Infirmary.'

'And you're a surgeon?'

'Yes, but I can turn my hand to most things when needed,' the doctor replied. 'I've been in this racket a long time. I was an army doctor for most of my career, but I do less cutting and more considering these days. I'm too long in the tooth to be amputating soldiers' limbs in dust-blown tents.'

'You don't think Jean has any problem understanding her situation?' Robert asked the doctor.

Dr Browne looked surprised. 'You'd know more about that than me, surely, Mr Kinniburgh? I can't even converse with the woman. To be honest, all I could tell from my examination was that she was physically healthy and not an obvious lunatic. I was hoping, when Sibbald told me you were likely to be here this morning, that you might assist me in assessing her mental state.'

'I see.' Despite the fact that he had formed a favourable impression of the doctor, Robert was unsure of this new development. He was in two minds as to whether he ought to help, given the doctor's earlier comments regarding Lord Succoth's option of incarceration in an asylum.

Dr Browne pressed him. 'I have one or two questions

147

that I am required to put to the prisoner. If you could convey them to her, I should be able to give a judgement to His Lordship. Otherwise, the lady is likely to remain in limbo for who knows how long.'

Robert weighed up his options.

'She cannot be kept locked up indefinitely, Mr Kinniburgh,' Dr Browne prompted.

'No,' Robert said, 'I suppose not. I will try my best to interpret for you.'

~

A few minutes later, Jean was conveyed back to the cell by the harried Sibbald. She busied herself adjusting her clothing, smoothing her bodice and fastening the cuffs of her blouse. She seemed surprised to find both Robert and Dr Browne in the cell and looked to Sibbald, as if for guidance. The keeper gestured to her to sit down at the table opposite Dr Browne and disappeared for a moment, returning with another chair for Robert.

Robert nodded a greeting to Jean and explained that Dr Browne had to ask a few more questions and he would interpret them for her. Sibbald stood at the fireplace watching them.

'How does your system work, Kinniburgh?' asked the doctor. 'Should I pose the first question to you?'

'Just speak normally,' explained Robert, 'as if I'm not here. All you need to do is pause after each sentence or so and I'll put your words into signs for Jean, then she'll answer by signs and I'll convey her meaning back to you.'

'Very well,' said the doctor, settling down to his task. 'Can I ask you, Miss Campbell, is there any history of lunacy in your family?'

Robert paused for a moment, considering how best to

sign *lunacy*. He had seen a variety of signs for madness. Some deaf people pointed at the side of their heads and indicated by a finger spiralling or a fist bursting that there was something broken inside a person's brain. Some used both hands to indicate some sort of agitation within the heart, a sign that was also used for anger. Robert decided to make signs related to the brain as he wanted Jean to be clear that the doctor was asking about her state of mind, rather than her distress at the situation she found herself in. He drew his palm behind his shoulder to indicate that Dr Browne was asking about the past, about any madness that might have existed in Jean's family.

Once she had understood the question, Jean snorted and Dr Browne, startled by the seeming inappropriateness of the prisoner's behaviour, looked back to Robert in bewilderment. Robert, concerned that the doctor would read Jean's behaviour as proof of madness rather than an expression of how ridiculous she felt the question was, immediately excused what Jean had done.

Suddenly, he was troubled by guilt; he was required to interpret, not to insinuate himself into the conversation.

He turned to face Jean.

Please. You must be serious, or it will go badly for you. Answer the doctor's question. Your family. Are any of them lunatics?

Jean shook her head adamantly. *No.* Robert relayed the answer and Dr Browne jotted something down in his notebook.

'Has she ever received treatment for lunacy or mental deficiency of any kind?' Dr Browne asked. 'Excepting being deaf and dumb, of course.'

Robert signed the question to Jean, resisting the urge to take exception to the doctor's inclusion of deafness in the gamut of mental sickness.

Again, Jean answered in the negative.

Browne then asked her to tell him if she had any of a series of symptoms that might indicate that she was not in her right mind. These included having violent thoughts, hearing voices, causing herself or others bodily harm, as well as a variety of obsessive habits. Jean calmly denied having any of these symptoms. Although, when Robert signed, *Do you hear voices?* they exchanged an incredulous glance.

Dr Browne, busy scribbling his answers down in his notebook, didn't notice.

When he came to the end of his list of questions, Dr Browne thanked Jean by copying the sign that Robert made and seemed immensely pleased with himself.

Jean drummed her hand on the table to gain Robert's attention.

He's asking me questions. Why?

He wants to know if you are mad or sane, Robert answered.

Why? she repeated.

If you're sane, they can take your case to court. If mad, they will take you to a hospital.

A madhouse?

Robert nodded.

Jean flushed with anger. *I'm not mad.*

I know.

Do you?

Yes.

Does he? Jean pointed at Dr Browne, who had been watching their exchange.

Robert said, 'Jean wants to know if you think she is mad or not?'

'She seems perfectly sane to me,' said the doctor. 'That's what I'll put in my report. A bit agitated, but I suppose that's to be expected.'

A bit agitated? Robert thought. It was no wonder. Still, they weren't about to cart Jean off to the asylum and for that he was grateful. He would have time to talk to her about what he had been up to in Glasgow. Perhaps, now that he had seen where she lived for himself, it might provide them with some common ground and help her to explain her story.

~

When both the doctor and Sibbald had left, Robert broached the original subject of his visit.

I'm sorry I haven't been here for a few days. I was in Glasgow.

Jean raised her eyebrows.

I went to visit the Deaf Church.

You saw the minister?

Robert nodded. *The minister and his wife. Also, their son. They made me very welcome.*

Jean nodded. *They are good people. Kind.*

They wanted to know how you are keeping. In this place.

Jean stood up suddenly. *I'm ashamed and wronged.* She turned to the wall, her back to Robert, and reached out her arms, rested her palms on the rough, cold stone. Her head bowed, she stood like that for what felt a long time. Robert couldn't tell if she was angry at him or simply frustrated by her imprisoned state. When she turned to face him, her eyes were filled with tears.

They keep well too? Jean asked.

Yes, Robert said. *They wish to help you, but they are as confused as I am about what happened.*

Robert watched her as she sat back down on the shabby wooden chair. A week ago, Jean had seemed at odds with this place, almost defiant. Now, the prisoner seemed to wear the mantle of her cell more easily, as if a bleaching had taken place and she had merged into the stonework. Or perhaps the bath that the doctor had procured for her had washed away more than sweat and dirt.

Robert continued. *I looked for Jim Donnelly, but I could not find him. He was not at his lodgings. His neighbours say he has gone away.*

Jean nodded. *He is often away. There is a weekly hiring fair. Sometimes he goes on a boat to work at the docks or with the teams that dig the canals.*

Robert sighed. *I spoke to a fair few people in Glasgow. No one had a good word to say about him.*

She shrugged. *That's the way of it, for the Irish.*

Robert raised his eyes to the ceiling. Every time he inched closer to the crime, Jean deflected attention from it by saying something practical or defensive.

I need you to tell me what happened to your baby. You have been charged with murder and protest your innocence of that charge. The man you suggest might be able to bolster your defence has gone missing and so there is no one who can say otherwise.

Jean looked at him with concern. *I'm sorry. Are you angry with me?*

I'm frustrated, that's what I am. I asked to visit Glasgow, but you gave me so little to go on that I worry I've wasted my time there.

Robert bristled. He felt the full indignation of someone who was being used. Who was using him and why, he found impossible to answer. Lord Succoth had sent him here. Did His Lordship know how difficult an undertaking this was? It wasn't the case itself but the prisoner who was difficult. Why did Jean behave in this obtuse manner? He had preferred her stories of Islay. They had a ring of truth. Whenever she was questioned about more recent events she dissembled. Perhaps he should stick to relaying her words truthfully rather than trying to find meaning. To tell the story. To fit the facts to his impressions of this woman.

I'm only charged with interpreting for you, Robert said. *You do understand that, don't you? I didn't need to go through to Glasgow. I could have stayed here. I'm a teacher. I could be teaching children that need my instruction.*

Go back to them then, Jean signed, abruptly. *It wasn't me that asked you to go all the way to Glasgow.*

Robert fought back the urge to point out her lack of gratitude for what he was trying to do. *Then you must accept your fate. Do you not rail against it? Perhaps you are lying to me.*

I am not lying, Jean countered, indignantly.

Robert regarded her steadily. *You are not telling the whole truth.*

He picked up his bag and greatcoat and walked towards the door of the cell.

Will you come back? Jean asked.

Robert thought for a moment before answering. *I don't know. If you will not speak the truth clearly to me, I can do no more than relay your words to the court. I can't, for the life of me, understand why that is enough for you. You are so adamant that you are innocent. That some other person harmed your baby. Why, then, do you not tell me who is guilty? If it is Jim Donnelly, you owe him no favours. He has upped and left with no thought for your predicament. I do not understand your loyalty. It is misplaced.*

Robert had said that he wasn't angry, but he could feel his fury building as he tried to convey to Jean how counterproductive her silence might be. She was weeping now, and he knew he ought to stop – to comfort her in some small way – but his frustrations continued to pour forth.

This couple you talk about, I cannot find them without a name. The Buchanans say they have no idea who they are. If you do not furnish me with more details, how can I plead your case? The events that you have made me aware of have no logic to them.

He closed his eyes and stood still for a moment.

Will you come back? she asked again.

Only if there is more you wish to tell me, Robert answered. *If not, I may as well just wait to see you in court. I'm not willing to waste my time going around in circles.*

I will tell you the truth.

Robert sighed. *Will you? It has been a long day for you. Have some food and rest over the weekend. Decide what you want to do. Send word by Sibbald and I will return. If you mean to tell your story. If not, leave me be.*

32

∼ Friday, 7 March 1817:
Chessels Court, Edinburgh ∼

After supper that evening, Robert retreated to his study with some of the older boys. The pupils were filled with excitement at the prospect of witnessing a balloon ascent by James Sadler. It had been announced in the newspaper that the great man would fly his balloon over Arthur's Seat and that the flight would take place on the first Saturday in April.

Robert had known about Sadler's proposed flight for many months now; the periodicals and journals his work enabled him to subscribe to were full of news of the Oxfordshire man's remarkable inventions and demonstrations.

In the schoolroom, Robert had used many of Sadler's exploits to illustrate concepts in science and mathematics. The older pupils were intrigued by Sadler's story and their infectious enthusiasm had spread throughout the school until even the younger children, with little or no understanding of the science behind his deeds, had become captivated by them. Margaret had encouraged them to draw pictures of hot air balloons flying over the city's landmarks.

Some considered James Sadler foolhardy, others thought him utterly insane, but Robert admired his scientific knowledge and his charisma and wanted to imbue his pupils with the enthusiasm and self-belief that this self-taught, sweet-shop boy had used to propel not only his balloons but his own career.

∼

Margaret shooed away the senior boys who were loitering in Robert's study, making it plain they should be in bed in readiness for another school day.

'And you're not much better than these daft boys, Robbie,' she said. 'You should have chased them long ago.'

'I'm sorry. I hadn't noticed the time.'

Margaret rolled her eyes.

'No wonder; you're too wrapped up in concern for your prisoner. You're still a schoolteacher, Robbie, the place can't run without you.'

'You and Isabella are doing a fine job, though,' said Robert. 'I am very grateful. You know that, don't you?'

'I do. But your gratitude is not enough. Isabella can take care of the girls and I can instruct the younger boys, but the older boys need you, Robbie. Look at Joseph – you've made him all kinds of promises about helping him with his sciences. He's keen to continue his studies and he's very able. I'd hate for him to miss out on a place because you've been too distracted when he needs you most.'

Robert looked aghast. 'How can you say that? We've just been discussing Sadler's balloon flight. I'm instructing Joseph in the fine details of how that's likely to be achieved and ensuring that he gets to experience the event for himself. There's no one more determined to help Joseph than me.'

'Where has that determination been for the last week? You've hardly been here. Until this evening, Joseph has been poring over his books all by himself. He's willing, Robbie, but he can't learn on his own, he needs you to explain things to him.'

'I will. This situation with Jean Campbell's case, it's temporary. Once I have done the groundwork and the case is given a trial date, things will start to return to how they were.'

Margaret walked over to the window and began drawing the curtains. She unhooked one length from a tasselled cord and gathered the expanse of heavy damask in the crook of her arm, before letting it fall to the ground. She patted the material down and arranged it very deliberately in equally spaced folds. The walls of Robert's study were tall, with a triple-fronted window that looked onto the enclosed central area of Chessels Court. Outside, a frost had crept over the pathway and was reaching out its fingers towards the steps that led to the main entrance to the school. The bare winter trees stood sentinel, patiently waiting for springtime to weave its warmth around them.

'I'm not sure we can simply go back to how things were, Robbie. Sometimes, we have to adapt to changes at an alarming rate. You might do better to concentrate on the central concerns of your life instead of frittering time away on the peripheries.'

Robert stacked his books neatly on his desk and screwed closed the lid of the jar of ink he had been using.

'What do you mean?'

'That you should choose which woman you spend your time with very carefully. That's all.'

'For goodness' sake, Maggie, I don't choose to spend time with Jean Campbell. This is my work, that's all.'

'You said yourself that she was attractive.'

'I did not. I said that I could see how someone might find her attractive, despite her disadvantages. I didn't say that I found her attractive. You're not being fair.'

He took his journal and placed it in the top drawer of the desk. He slammed it hard as he did so and immediately regretted this show of emotion.

'Are you jealous?' he asked, irritably.

'Of course not,' Margaret snapped, 'What a ridiculous thing to say. I'm tired, Robbie.'

She turned and made for the door.

'Wait. Don't leave,' Robert said. 'I'm sorry if I've been neglecting you. I know it's not easy doing the work of two people.'

'No,' said Margaret, 'it's not. I have things to talk to you about and no time in which to do it.'

'I don't have to go to the Tolbooth over the weekend. Perhaps we could have some time alone? I could carry on here for a couple of hours and get some more work out of the way. Then I would be able to devote the whole of Saturday and Sunday to my family and my pupils.'

'I don't know,' Margaret said, flatly. 'It would be a start, I suppose.'

~

Margaret was still awake when Robert came to bed, but she lay still, not willing to initiate another conversation. Robert crept around in the dark, divesting himself of his clothes and pulling on his nightshirt. He shivered as he felt around for the edge of the bed and got inside and pulled the blankets over him.

'Are you awake?' he asked.

'Yes.'

'Maggie, I know a school isn't the best place for privacy. There is much to be done. We can get out early on Sunday, go to church and then have time to ourselves for a few hours.'

'Yes, let's run away from our duties,' she said, shortly. 'I don't imagine they'll still be waiting for us when we get back. Perhaps the fairies will see to them.'

Robert sighed, determined not to pour oil on troubled waters. 'If it was up to me, we would have private quarters where we could have a separate family life, but the business of the school, the running of it and the finding of money to continue running it, it seems to take up so much time.'

'I know.'

'I do love you, Maggie.'

'I know.'

'Are you to give any more than two-syllable answers this night?'

'I shouldn't think so.'

'That was five syllables.'

'Top marks for arithmetic, Robbie.'

'I don't want us to argue.'

'Well, stop provoking me.'

'Very well.'

Robert turned to her and moved his arm, wrapping it tentatively around her waist.

Margaret sighed.

'Is that too provoking?' asked Robert.

'No.' Margaret relaxed, and Robert moved his body towards her. She curled into him and sighed again.

'Will you sing me a song?' he asked.

Margaret laughed incredulously. 'Will I sing you a song? I thought you were after something else entirely! What kind of song?'

'A sad song,' said Robert. 'That one about the girls building a house.'

'"Bessie Bell and Mary Gray"? Is that the one you mean?'

'I think so.'

'Oh, very well.' Margaret turned over to lie on her back and began to sing, and Robert lay on his side, listening in the darkness.

33

∾ Sunday, 9 March 1817:
Edinburgh Castle ∾

It was still the forenoon when Robert and Margaret turned into Mound Place and began to climb up the vertiginous hill that led through the New College in the direction of the castle. They had risen early on this particular Sunday and attended an early service at church so that they could pass some time in each other's company before returning to school and beginning preparations for the evening meal.

The sharp, sheer corner on this approach to the castle was always a challenge and, although Robert pressed on, Margaret was grateful to reach an iron handrail that was secured to the east wall.

'Robbie,' Margaret called to her husband, 'can we not stop for a wee minute?'

Her voice was lost in a rush of wind that barrelled down from the Royal Mile towards the valley below. Robert was just a few steps in front of her and, when he turned around to check her progress, he read her meaning in the expression on her face. He shook his head, in mock outrage at her giving up so soon, and she laughed and stamped her foot like a petulant child. Robert slowed down, retraced his last few steps and came to a halt beside her.

There was no one else on the street and Robert put his arm around her shoulders and pulled her to him. They stumbled for a second and then embraced on the windy corner.

From where they stood, the road dipped rapidly down

towards the Nor Loch and from hence, meadows stretched all the way to the Firth of Forth, a landscape dotted with hamlets of loosely grouped cottages and the odd large estate house. To the north-east lay Leith, with its jumble of ships' masts crowded into its small harbour.

The sea was a broad blue sword, splitting the Lothians from the Fifeshire coast. A raft of clouds hung heavy like rows of billowed sheets ready to be folded. In the foreground, machines and plant stood idle – no work being undertaken on a Sunday. At the far side of the Nor Loch, stakes had been hammered into the ground, and ran the length of the south bank. The city was in the process of being redrawn – an orderly grid in the manner of that at Bath had been promised to Edinburgh's denizens. Rows of elegant, light buildings with expansive roads and gardens would be an antidote to the medieval crush of the steps and vennels that emitted from the skeleton of the High Street. As yet, this ideal creation existed only as a sketch in progress – to the untrained eye there were nothing but tentative brushstrokes in piles of earth and gaping trenches. The newspapers talked of architectural competitions and the ordered delights of a grid-like plan of housing and commerce; a release from the cheek-by-jowl existence in the old town. Neither Robert nor Margaret could envisage the completion of such a thing. There were plans to drain the Nor Loch and harness the power of the new railways but even this, though promised, seemed bizarre and outlandish.

On this clear Sabbath morning, the merging of sea and meadow and sky was a picture so perfect that an artist of repute could not better it, and the Kinniburghs were chock-full of hope and gratitude.

Margaret slipped her fingers between Robert's. 'I have something to tell you, Robbie,' she said.

Absent-mindedly, Robert pulled her close, his eyes still trained on the coastline. 'What is it?'

'Would you be interested in becoming a father at all?'

Robert wasn't really following what she was saying. For her part, Margaret was taut with foreknowledge and desperate for Robert to latch on to the importance of what she was hinting at.

'What?' he said again.

'Oh, for pity's sake, Robbie, I'm going to have a baby.'

He stood awkwardly for a second, not sure how to react, having never been told he was to be a father before.

'I'm glad,' he said. 'A bit apprehensive, if I'm honest, but glad. Are you well?'

'Very well, thank you.'

Then, he folded her body into his and they stood on the corner for a long time.

They walked up to the esplanade at the castle, the midday sun of winter alternately blinding them and then deserting them as it keeked through gaps in the buildings.

34

~ *Sunday, 9 March 1817:*
Chessels Court, Edinburgh ~

Robert was in his study. A half-drunk glass of brandy sat beside the open book of scripture on his desk that he was not reading. He was thinking about Jean and wrestling with his recent behaviour at the Tolbooth. Given the circumstances, it was wholly understandable that he had admitted his frustration, but he couldn't shake the feeling that he had behaved like an ill-tempered child and it was not to his credit.

He gazed at the triptych framed by the study windows. The dark, bare landscape suited his mood. Branches of trees shifted against a charcoal sky. Everything was indistinct in the gloom.

A shape moved suddenly amidst the trees and startled him. As it came nearer, he realised that it was a man. Robert watched the man approach the front door and heard the rattle of the knocker against its plate. Isabella's bedroom was on the ground floor. He heard her footsteps hurry towards the lobby and open the door, his sister-in-law's soft voice contrasting with a rougher tongue. Robert got up from the desk and went to find out who the visitor was.

He was surprised to see Thomas Sibbald standing in the hallway. The collar of the keeper's greatcoat was turned up against the cold and the swift removal of his hat had made his scant hair stand up on end.

'Mr Sibbald,' he said, 'is everything alright?' Robert felt

his stomach lurch, suddenly worried that Jean had done something foolish.

'Fine, sir,' Sibbald replied. 'I was just telling Miss Menzies, here, I've come with a message. I'm sorry to disturb you so late in the evening, but the prisoner, Campbell, was quite insistent that I ask you to come to the Tolbooth.'

'Now?' Robert asked. 'Can it not wait until morning?'

'I don't believe so, sir. The prisoner wishes you to return as soon as possible. She seems to have something of import to relate.'

'Well, Mr Sibbald, that might be the case, but Jean Campbell has had ample opportunity to let me into her confidence since I first met her last week and, frankly, it's been like pulling teeth to get a straight answer out of her.'

Isabella looked at him askance and Robert felt the need to justify his irritation.

'I'm fast losing patience, man, and now she chooses the Sabbath to click her fingers and summon me? Who's to say she won't clam up again when I return to the cell?'

Sibbald shifted uneasily. 'I understand your vexation, Mr Kinniburgh, but I'd be very grateful if you might give her this chance. If it proves fruitless, I'll not ask again. You have my word.'

Robert shook his head. 'It's not your word that I doubt; you're only doing your duty.'

'Even so, you have it,' Sibbald repeated.

Robert sighed. 'Wait a minute,' he said. 'I'll fetch my things and come along with you.'

He turned to his sister-in-law, who was watching this exchange with curiosity.

'Can you tell Maggie that I've had to go out? I don't know when I'll be back.'

'Of course, Robert. Good luck.'

'Aye, I'll need it.'

The two men strode quickly in the direction of the Tolbooth. The streets were quiet, little traffic was abroad and only the travellers' inns emanated any noise. The dispossessed who habitually wandered Edinburgh's night-time thoroughfares were tucked into doorways in search of shelter and what warmth the cold stone could offer them. The High Street was patrolled by constables who were apt to prod bundles roughly with their sticks, so those who slept on the capital's streets tended to slip off into alleyways and closes to hunker down for the night.

When they reached the Tolbooth, Sibbald took out his set of keys and let them in by the back door. The central stairway was poorly lit, and Robert had to concentrate on negotiating the worn, well-trodden steps, keeping a protective grip on the banister as he climbed upwards to Jean's cell.

So Sibbald had left the prison unattended, Robert thought. That was a risk to take. As far as Robert was aware, the keeper could be summarily dismissed if he deserted his post. It was dangerous to leave prisoners alone, albeit under lock and key.

35

~ *Sunday, 9 March 1817:*
The Tolbooth Prison, Edinburgh ~

It's near midnight, Robert began. He perched at the windowsill, reluctant to commit himself to a chair. *If you have something to tell me, I suggest that you start now. I'm not at your beck and call.*

I know, Jean replied.

Robert pointed to a space directly in front of him. *The truth is here,* he signed, using his index finger as a signifier. Finally, he pointed at Jean. *You circle around it, keeping it hidden.* Robert raised both palms, sliding one behind the other. *You say you are not a fool, but you play at one when it suits you. I believe you have a choice. Firstly, you can put on a dumb show, reflect back what these men assume of your character. Perhaps they will feel pity for you and let you walk free? That would be a risk. They could just as easily regard you as a lunatic and lock you up.*

Jean seemed confused. *The doctor doesn't think I'm mad.*

Robert sighed. *The doctor only gives an opinion. If it suits the court to think you a lunatic, they will override his evidence. You know how often the deaf are misunderstood. It would take very little for them to connect deafness to madness.* He curled his thumbs and forefingers into circles and looped them together to make a chain.

She pursed her lips and stretched out her hands in the manner of a set of weighing scales. *You said there was a choice?*

Yes, he continued, *you can give me evidence that proves your innocence in your child's murder. To do this, you must be open with me.*

And if that puts me in danger?

You are to be tried for murder. There is every chance you will hang. How much more danger can you possibly be in?

If they find out about the bargain I made?

The bargain was never settled. You have no money from these people. I can't deny it was wrong, but it was done for the right reasons.

You said Jim is gone. I don't know where Sandy is. I need to make sure he is safe and looked after.

Could he be with your aunt and uncle? I can send a letter to the Reverend Buchanan asking him to find out on your behalf.

Please. Jean looked up at him. *I don't worry for myself. I can't bear to think of him on the streets or locked up in the poorhouse. He is too young to fend for himself.*

Robert rolled his shoulders back and stretched. Tiredness and the chill night air that hung heavy within the cell had crept into his bones and he felt a need to move around, to alleviate the physical pressure he felt, if nothing else.

I will make my own bargain with you. If you tell me tonight what I need to know to help you avoid prison or worse, I will find out where Sandy is and make sure he's looked after.

Jean nodded.

If I think you are hiding anything, I will walk away, and I will not return. I will interpret your signs in the courtroom and no more. Do you understand? I have nothing to lose. I'm not the one being put on trial here.

I understand, she acknowledged.

Then perhaps you might tell me why your baby died when it fell from that bridge.

My baby was already dead by the time I was on the bridge, Jean said.

167

Robert stiffened. *I'm sorry. How did your child come to die?*

He was killed in the house to the west of the city.

Robert looked astonished. He asked Jean to repeat what she had signed to make sure he understood her correctly.

Can you explain this to me?

It is a long story.

I have time enough to listen.

~

Robert warmed his hands on a cup of weak tea and watched as Sibbald busied himself blowing on the embers of the fire that had been banked a few hours ago. Once he had coaxed the fire back to life, the keeper wedged the cell door open while he swept the landing and stairway.

The scene was decidedly odd, thought Robert. It was almost as if the Tolbooth were no longer operating as a place of incarceration. Sibbald was becoming more like an innkeeper than a gaoler with each day that passed. God knew what the authorities would say if they could see this casual, laissez-faire attitude to the cold-blooded child killer that they must surely have read about in the papers.

I know it's difficult, Robert said, reaching out and touching Jean's hand, *but please, try to tell me what happened in the house.*

Jean sighed. *I don't know where to begin. Everything is mixed up in my mind.*

Robert smiled weakly. *I understand. I will try to help you. We can do this together. Why don't you begin by telling me something of their house?*

She nodded. *The day I arrived, Jim said goodbye at the gate, and I walked up to the front door. I rang the bell, and, after a few moments, a girl answered it. I didn't know what*

168

to do because I'd thought the man would answer. I didn't know how to explain who I was to this girl, so I smiled at her and made a sign to show I was deaf. You know the way you do when you don't think they'll understand you?

Jean showed Robert this sign, tapping her ear and shaking her head.

The girl looked me up and down and started smiling too. She seemed to know who I was. She led me first into a hallway and then to a large room where she pointed at a chair and asked me to sit down. I felt very strange in such a place, but the girl was kind and made a gesture that I supposed was her asking if I wanted a drink, so I nodded, and she went out of the room. In a few moments she came back with a teapot and a cup and poured it out for me.

Robert concentrated as Jean told the story. He could see that it would have been unexpected indeed for someone of her social station to have been invited in to such a house and treated as if she belonged there.

Jean resumed, *The door opened again, and the man came in. Full of welcoming smiles and making such a fuss of me. He tried to use some signs. Unlike the girl, he knew how to say hello and ask how I was; I assumed he had come across them at the Deaf Church. He was showing off to the girl. She smiled at him – not the way she had to me – more out of duty, I thought.*

You got the impression that she didn't like him? Robert asked.

I wasn't sure. Not then. He seemed very pleased with himself.

The corners of Jean's mouth turned down, suggesting her distaste.

He spoke to the girl and then made some more signs to me; that I should finish my tea and then the girl would show me to my room and give me something to eat if I was hungry.

Jean gestured towards a low table. *May I have a drink?*

Robert poured from a jug of small beer and handed a mug over to her.

I was left alone. Later, the girl – the maid – came back and took me to my bedroom, upstairs. It was in the attic, next to her own room. A bed and a washstand, with a window in the roof that looked up to the sky. I set down my reticule and shawl on the bed and we both went down to the kitchen.

Was the maid the only servant in the house? asked Robert.

Jean shook her head. *There was an older woman in the kitchen. She did the cooking and some of the other chores. There was a gardener who came once or twice while I was there. Only the maid lived in the house.*

Did you meet the mistress when you arrived?

The next day. She showed me to a nursery, just along from where they themselves slept. It was beautiful. There was a cradle, covered in white cotton, ribboned and tied to the frame. And a soft mattress and pillows in it. I couldn't believe my baby would sleep in such comfort. There were toys along a mantelpiece and picture books on some shelves. I used to look at them after the baby was born, when I was feeding him.

And you gave birth to your baby there?

Jean nodded.

There was a bed in the room and that was where I had my baby. Some days after I arrived. Around three weeks.

36

∼ Thursday, 30 January 1817:
Partickhill Road, Glasgow ∼

Jean was in the kitchen, having a cup of tea, when the nausea began to rise in her throat. She took another sip of the sugary tea to try to quell it but that only made it worse.

Ina peered at her from the opposite side of the table.

Martha was scrubbing down the bunkers in the pantry.

'Is she alright, do you think, hen?' Ina shouted through to Martha.

The housemaid stopped what she was doing and came directly. She crouched down beside Jean and patted the deaf woman's hand.

'Are you sick?' she mouthed at her, clutching at her own stomach and miming a retching motion. Then turning to Ina, in a completely unnecessary whisper, 'She's awfy white, do you not think?'

Jean stood up abruptly, holding a hand up to them both as if to say leave me alone, I'm fine, I'll sort myself out. She stumbled through the scullery door, in search of the privy.

The McDougalls kept a necessary house a few yards from the back door, on a cinder path that led to a jumble of outbuildings tucked behind the villa's uniform front facade. Jean groped her way along in the dark and fumbled for the latch.

Once inside, she pushed her hair back from her face and leant over the opening to the waste pit below. She retched two or three times, despairing of any release, but eventually a stream of liquid vomit came. She sat on the ground and breathed slowly, trying to collect herself. She felt marginally better, although her throat felt rough, and her muscles strained.

She wanted the lavatory now. She hitched up her dress, pulled down her drawers and perched on the rough wooden seat. Almost as soon as she sat down, shit came out of her in a torrent and splattered onto the earth below. She felt an odd pulling sensation in her groin followed by an emptying, and she recognised the signs. There were no real contractions as yet, and what had come out of her was too far down in the pit to examine, even if she had been of a mind to, but she was sure that the plug had been dislodged from its stopper and it was now just a matter of time before her pains began.

Jean cast about beside her for something to wipe herself with and her fingers alighted on a pile of leaves left in the necessary for that purpose. She hitched up her drawers again and righted herself as best she could in the dark, cramped surroundings.

When she flicked the latch and opened the door, she almost knocked Martha over. The housemaid had been sent out to keep an eye on her. As Jean stepped out of the necessary house, the wind blew the door open, and its edge caught Martha on the leg. Martha hopped up and down swearing and rubbing at her shin; Jean was distraught at having hurt the girl. Once the bolt to the lavatory was secured, they both shambled along the path into the light of the kitchen.

'All you've got is a skint knee, Martha Sproull,' Ina tutted, as she peeled off the girl's stocking and took a damp cloth from the sink to bathe it. 'Stop greeting and let me look at it.'

'It's nipping,' Martha said.

Jean patted the girl's arm. She made a fist and moved it in a circle at her chest. *I'm sorry, I didn't mean to hurt you.* Martha got the gist of it from Jean's disconsolate expression.

'Right,' Ina asserted, 'now we've patched you up, can we find out if all's well with Jean?'

Martha adopted the aspect of a brave soldier.

Jean, however, was righted for now and waved away Ina's concern, taking herself off to bed and promising to alert Martha if anything else should occur.

37

~ Friday, 31 January 1817:
Partickhill Road, Glasgow ~

Jean woke before daybreak. A dragging sensation in her back and an unaccountable restlessness already settled upon her. She felt tired and wished she could have remained asleep, building up her strength for the labour she knew was around the corner.

She got out of bed and drew her shawl around her shoulders. It was made of angora wool, a dark blue colour. It was one of a pair that Martha had given to her on her arrival, along with a further three full sets of clothes. Soft as it was, she missed her old plaid shawl and wished it hadn't been taken away.

Jean began to pace the narrow room, propelled by an inexplicable instinct for movement. It helped, though, to take her mind off the dull ache in her belly.

After a while, she stopped at the small window, looking down at Partick from her elevated vantage point. The sky was layered in dark greys and blues, like the folds of an organza dress. A splinter of coral pink hinted at the day yet to come.

She smoothed the curve of her belly under her nightgown and held it from underneath. The baby had stopped moving as much. For the last few weeks, it had wriggled and kicked and flipped like a fish, until she had grown demented with it. Now, it lay quiet, biding its time.

Her pains began as the day established itself. Jean

watched as the sun began to burn through an expanse of grey cloud until only white streams and patches were left on the blue. Beyond the garden wall were green fields that swept down towards the buildings of Partick and the river beyond. Rows of spindly young trees had been planted, delineating the borders between properties. A tabby cat that practically matched the mottled stone of a wall got up from a patch of moss, stretched and rearranged itself into an almost identical position as the one it had left.

The cramps, which had started as an indeterminate ache in her back, slowly crept around and encircled her belly. The idea of grappling with stays and clasps and buttons depressed her beyond measure, so she remained in her nightclothes and began to tidy the already pristine room. She smoothed the linen on the bed, tucking the corners of the sheets neatly under the mattress. She opened a deep drawer in the tallboy and took out a clean nightdress – releasing from a muslin bag a scent of lavender that permeated the room – and laid it down on the bed for later. The nightdress she was currently wearing would have to be boil washed by the time this was over. Perhaps they would burn it, she thought, erase the traces of her even while she remained in their house.

Her contractions were still mercifully brief by the time Martha waved a handkerchief through the partially open bedroom door and Jean ushered the girl inside the room. This was a method of communication that Martha had invented and of which she was inordinately proud. Every morning, she would bring Jean's breakfast upstairs on a tray. The house still asleep, Martha liked to have a few moments in Jean's company before it was time to lay out bread and jam and a pot of tea for the master and mistress.

A sudden pain gripped Jean as Martha was setting down a plate and a cup on the bedside table. The girl was startled by Jean's howl of pain and left off her task to bid Jean sit down on the bed. Martha leant her forward and rubbed at the small of her back.

She held Jean's upper arm and turned to face her.

The doctor? Martha asked, tapping two fingers to her wrist as if she were taking someone's pulse. *Will I fetch him now?*

Jean shook her head emphatically and gave a smile of reassurance.

Will we wait for Ina? Martha made a sign as if she were beating batter in a bowl to indicate that she meant the cook and housekeeper.

Jean nodded. She had no desire to be attended to by Dr Wilson, but she knew that McDougall would insist upon it. He was the type of man, after all, that set great store by the abilities of his fellows. Even the ineffectual Wilson could be trusted more than a bunch of women to bring his child into the world. Jean didn't trust the doctor to find his own arse with a map and was content to wait until Ina arrived to begin work or to muddle through herself with Martha's help.

While she had no qualms about assisting with the birth, and was perfectly confident that she and Jean could do it together, Martha was wary of going against the master's wishes. In the streets that she came from, babies were often born healthy, and mothers recovered soon enough. There was a period of intense labour and then it was over. Everyone ended up tired but happy. Of course, occasionally a baby failed to thrive, or a mother acquired an affliction from which she never recovered, but that was to be expected. She had heard some terrible stories from her mother and her friends about the intervention of doctors and the consequences for the women involved. Doctors cost money, so they weren't much in evidence in Castlebank

Street. Men, according to Martha's mother, were generally worse than useless and best kept away from birthing, so why anyone would get a doctor in, even if they could afford it, was beyond Martha's ken.

~

When Ina arrived, the dirty dishes were still on the kitchen table. Usually, by this hour, Martha would have taken them to the scullery, washed, dried and put them away. This morning, the teapot was cold, the cosy lying beside it, spent tealeaves pooled in the bottom of the cups.

As Ina was tying her pinny, Martha hurried through the kitchen door.

'Are you alright, hen?' Ina asked.

'Aye, I'm fine,' Martha replied. 'It's Jean. The baby is on the way. She wants you to come upstairs.'

Ina took a deep breath. 'Has the doctor been called for?'

'No,' Martha said, shamefacedly. 'Jean disnae want the doctor.'

Ina said, 'Aye, well, it's no really for Jean to say, hen.'

Ina busied herself collecting cloths and towels to take upstairs. 'Right, you away outside and draw some water. Is the master in?'

Martha shook her head. 'No. He went to his work half an hour ago.'

Ina raised an eyebrow. 'And he disnae know Jean's reached her time?'

Martha shook her head again.

'And the mistress?'

Another shake of the head.

'Well, it's gonnae get gey noisy in a wee while. She'll have to be told.'

'Can you no do it?' asked Martha. 'I'm feart she'll be angry with me.'

Ina sighed. 'Aye, I suppose so. You get that water now and bring it up to the bedroom. After that, you're going to have to get that doctor or we'll both be for the high jump.'

Ina bustled out of the kitchen and Martha stood for a second, a rising panic at her breast.

~

When Martha brought up a pail of water, Ina told her to set it down by the end of the bed. Jean was holding on to the bedstead with both of her hands, breathing heavily. Ina stroked the deaf woman's hair back from her face and wiped the sweat off her forehead.

'It's alright, hen,' she mouthed. 'I need to tell the mistress. We'll likely need to get the doctor to you.' Ina made a sign, two fingers tapping at the veins in her wrist. A sign that she'd learnt from Jean. 'I'm sorry,' Ina mouthed, shaking her head to signify regret.

It didn't matter now. Jean was pacing the room, waiting for the next contraction, oblivious to anything other than her own labour.

Ina told Martha to turn down the bedclothes and wait with Jean until she got back from seeing the mistress. The old cook went along the corridor and knocked on Euphemia's bedroom door. When she returned, she told Martha to get her coat on and run down to Dr Wilson's house.

'What did the mistress say?' Martha asked.

'Nothing for you to worry about hen, she's wired to the moon that one. It'll take more than this to rouse her. You, just away and do as you're told. I can look after Jean until you get back.'

Jean made a noise like an animal growling in pain and Ina tilted her face to look at her directly. Ina began to make short breaths and encouraged Jean to copy her. Martha was on her way out of the room, but the cook shouted after her to come back.

'I think we'll have to do this ourselves, hen,' said Ina., 'There's no time to get the doctor before Jean's baby arrives. Go to the corner and pay that auld cawdie to take a message to Wilson; tell him that he's to get here as soon as he's able.'

Ina sat with Jean and, when Martha returned, they both got the deaf woman onto the bed and began spreading towels beneath her, hitching up her nightdress to let her knees fall apart. Martha dipped a sponge in the pail of water and handed it to Jean, who squeezed it across her shoulders and onto her chest, thankful of the cooling sensation. Ina pushed up the window to let some air in.

~

The pains were coming thick and fast now. Ina rolled up her sleeves, looking for all the world like she was about to joint a rabbit. As Jean groaned into each contraction, Martha held her hand, willing her through it. Soon the crown of the baby's head was visible, slick and dark against the pale skin of its mother's thighs. Jean grimaced through another contraction and one bony shoulder juddered forth, splattering the towels and bedclothes in blood-streaked membrane. Another shoulder and, all at once, the baby tumbled out in a mass of limbs and fluid.

For a few seconds, time seemed to suspend itself while Ina and Martha gazed at the wee marvel in front of them. The baby lay frigid and still, as if the shock of coming into the world had been too much to bear. Then, all at once, it let out an almighty howl. Ina swept the wee one up in a clean towel.

'A boy,' she mouthed.

Jean smiled as the older woman handed him over. She clasped the wee fellow to her breast and looked at him with such joy that Martha was transfixed by the beauty of it. A new life brought forth. A commonplace miracle. It was, at that moment, as if they were the only people that were truly alive and conscious of God's presence.

Then the front doorbell sounded.

'I'll get it, hen,' Ina said. 'You stay here.'

A few moments later, the front door opened; footsteps hurried up the stairs and Martha remembered that this was not only a beginning but an ending.

38

∾ Monday, 10 March 1817:
Adam Square, Edinburgh ∾

'Can we establish that we are all in agreement, gentlemen?'

Lord Succoth addressed the trio of men sitting in his drawing room. Along with Robert were Dr Edwin Browne and a rather fey academic, Jeremiah Pringle, Professor of Moral Philosophy at the University of Edinburgh. Succoth had invited all three to join him in the early evening to make a final decision regarding Jean's ability to plead. They were gathered around another of the house's vast fireplaces, where warm flames crackled and reflected in the pale grey marble of its surround.

Robert fiddled with his glass of port and hoped that one of his two companions would answer Succoth's question first. True to form, the no-nonsense medical man, Edwin Browne, proffered an opinion.

'I'm happy to certify her physically fit, Your Lordship,' Dr Browne asserted. 'There's no reason to think that the prisoner has any mental incapacity beyond her inability to hear proceedings and, from what I've seen, Mr Kinniburgh appears more than able to surmount that difficulty.'

Succoth nodded. 'And yourself, Professor Pringle, do you concur with this viewpoint?'

Robert had never met Pringle before this evening, but he had long known of him by reputation. Of the three men who had been asked for their opinion by Lord Succoth, Professor Pringle had been the first of them to meet and examine Jean Campbell. In fact, it had been the professor who had recommended that someone be brought in to interpret for the prisoner when he found he was not able to communicate with her.

Pringle adopted a pained expression that Robert suspected, was self-consciously designed to suggest that the case he was considering was a particularly complicated one that he alone could be trusted to disentangle.

'From an intellectual point of view, the prisoner doesn't seem to differ particularly from those of her sex and class who have the ability to hear. If Mr Kinniburgh feels confident that he has the means to convey her testimony to the court, then I see no reason why the trial cannot go ahead.'

'Professor, do you believe the deaf and dumb are able to understand the concept of right and wrong?' asked Succoth.

'I'd go further,' Pringle said. 'I think there is every reason to believe them capable of finer feelings than those experienced by the rest of society.'

Succoth looked confused. 'Can you explain what you mean by that, Professor?'

Pringle nodded. 'If someone is deprived of one of their senses, those that are left increase to fill the vacuum. It follows that this amplification of remaining senses can only lead to a greater amount of consciousness on the part of the deaf and dumb.'

Robert suppressed a groan. He had heard this 'savant' notion advanced elsewhere from time to time but had little patience for it. It seemed to him that, with regard to the deaf, society was divided into those who looked down upon them as little more than grotesques and those who elevated them to the status of saints by dint of their silent martyrdom. While the latter attitude resulted in less harsh treatment, neither seemed to chime with his own experience of deaf people being as disparate as everyone else.

Succoth, however, seemed intrigued by Pringle's hypothesis, which was a surprise to Robert who, up until now, had thought His Lordship entirely disinterested in Jean's deafness.

'When you talk of finer feelings, what exactly do you mean?' Succoth asked the professor. 'Physical sensation or emotions, for example?'

Pringle's brow furrowed again. 'I would categorise them as cerebral feelings or notions that are gleaned by the heart or intellect. Nothing to do with the corporeal as such.'

Succoth again looked confused. 'How does that theory relate to this crime?' he asked. 'She threw the baby in the river. That's not disputed.'

'A baby was reported as having fallen into the river,' Robert interjected. 'Whether it happened or if Jean threw it in or not hasn't been established.'

'Aye, well, that will be for the jury to decide,' said Succoth. 'I can't see how the panel's finer feelings will be relevant.'

Professor Pringle appeared to be gearing up for further discussion, but Succoth cut in abruptly.

'So, if we're all happy to proceed, the trial will go ahead next week. I'll have my clerk take the necessary steps and keep you all informed.'

His Lordship stood up abruptly.

'Thank you for your work so far, gentlemen, it's much appreciated. However, I must away. I have another engagement this evening.'

~

When they left, Professor Pringle sped off in the direction of the university and Robert and Dr Browne walked east from Lord Succoth's residence. Dr Browne was headed for his rooms near Surgeon's Hall and Robert was content to join him before pressing on down through the Canongate towards the Deaf and Dumb Institution.

'You're not persuaded that Jean Campbell is guilty, are you?' Browne asked as they crossed over onto Infirmary Street.

'In all honesty, I'm convinced she's innocent,' Robert replied. 'I just don't know how to prove it.'

'Who could have killed her baby if not herself?' Edwin asked. 'She was seen to throw it from the bridge, was she not?'

'Jean maintains a couple intended to adopt the baby, but something went wrong.'

'I see,' said Edwin, 'Have this couple been traced?'

Robert sighed, 'No. I need their name and Jean does not have it to give me. She has tried to describe where they live and how she first came into contact with the husband but the only other person who can connect them to her is Jean's common-law husband, and he is nowhere to be found. I intend to return to Glasgow. I wish I were better connected in that city; if I can only identify these people, she would stand more of a chance of justice.'

'You'll need evidence if you are to save her, Robert,' said Edwin. 'Succoth is only interested in hard facts. I'm surprised Succoth is funding another visit to Glasgow. He's not usually so free with the public purse.'

'He doesn't know,' Robert admitted.

Edwin raised his eyebrows in confusion.

'I'm going to Glasgow to give a demonstration of the methods we use at the institution,' he explained.

They continued in silence for some moments.

'Have you ever attended the High Court?' asked Edwin. Robert shook his head.

'I've given expert testimony at many trials,' Edwin

continued. 'They're not occasions that take much account of nuance. They deal in right or wrong and the jury makes their decision based purely on what is placed in front of them on the day. Once again: you'll need hard facts.'

39

~ Tuesday, 11 March 1817:
Calton, Glasgow ~

Robert sat on one of two hoop-backed chairs that had been placed at the front of the church. A low table with a jug of water and two glasses had been stationed between the chairs. He watched attentively as people were directed to their seats by the minister and his wife, feeling slightly self-conscious of the curious glances in his direction.

Although he felt bone-weary after his journey on the early stage from Edinburgh, Robert couldn't help but be pleasantly surprised at the level of interest in his presentation. Despite his self-effacing manner, Angus Buchanan was obviously well connected in the city.

As each pew filled, some of the men were forced to give up their seats as more ladies arrived. Folk stood to the side and at the back of the small church, holding on to the ends of pews or leaning on the rough plaster walls. There were married couples and small groups made up of merchants and tradesmen, their wives and families. Well-to-do citizens kitted out in expensive suits and gowns. The merchants were self-made men who earned their money through the movement of commodities around the globe. The tradesmen used their skills to build the premises that housed these commodities as well as erecting the secular, civic halls in which the merchants invested their money and sought to expand their power and influence.

At the front of the church, two pews were taken up

solely by members of Angus Buchanan's deaf congregation. On Robert's instruction, the minister had ensured that they were all grouped together. The deaf people sat unusually still, conscious that Robert had asked them to desist from signing to each other until he began his presentation. Now and then, one or other of them would turn around to look at the strangers who packed into their humble place of worship.

When the door to the church closed, Angus called the assembly to order.

'Fellow Christians, welcome to our church. I am delighted that so many have made the journey here this evening to hear about the tremendous work being done by my friend from Edinburgh; teacher to those to whom the Lord has given an affliction to be borne bravely. Please, extend a hearty welcome to Mr Robert Kinniburgh.'

A ripple of applause echoed around the small church.

'Mr Kinniburgh,' Angus continued, 'has been good enough to make a second visit to Glasgow in as many weeks and we are fortunate indeed that he has seen fit to spend some time with our congregation.'

Robert stood up and both signed and spoke his thanks to Angus. He faced the portion of his audience that contained the deaf parishioners and at once began to sign.

I am very happy to be back in the city of Glasgow and I am glad that your minister has invited me to talk to you this evening. I am a teacher, master at the Deaf and Dumb Institution in Edinburgh and, this evening, I will share some stories about the children under my supervision, the new educational methods we employ and the happier, more useful future that I see for deaf people in Scotland.

The deaf people concentrated on Robert's signs, a few being unfamiliar to them. Most nodded and smiled to indicate that they understood the gist of his message.

The hearing people in the congregation stole surreptitious glances at them.

Robert carried on. He asked Angus to hold up one of his pamphlets and he pointed at the illustration on the front cover.

This is a picture of our school. It was drawn by my wife. We have almost fifty pupils at the moment. They are of different ages up to fifteen years old and come mostly from Scotland, although we have a few from further afield in England and even across the water in Ireland. Nearly all of them are boarders at the school. Those whose families have the means pay for some or all of their upkeep. A few others have their fees paid by their local parish or by a private benefactor or a mixture of these.

Again, the deaf people he addressed followed his speech with interest. This time, however, some of the hearing folk began to get restless. They made up the majority of the audience and yet here was Mr Kinniburgh conversing solely with the deaf and dumb.

The Reverend Buchanan had invited them along to hear of the efficiency of this man's institution. They had been expecting to see an exhibition of his methods and be induced to subscribe to the enterprise. Their patronage would go to a class of individuals from whom God had withheld the blessings of sound and speech and yet here they were being made to feel excluded; it was perhaps not the best method of getting them to part with their money.

Robert was well aware of their feelings and yet he did nothing to stop this sense of unease from permeating the room. At last, he nodded his thanks to the group of deaf people and turned his attention to the company at large.

'I hope you'll excuse me. I do not intend to give any

offence. I gave the Reverend Buchanan my word that I would both speak and sign this evening. However, I didn't tell him which method of communication I would begin with.'

Robert raised his eyebrows and murmurs of tentative laughter could be heard from some sections of the audience.

Robert gestured to a group of ladies in the front pew, their straw bonnets tied beneath their chins with ribbons of various colours.

'May I ask a favour of you, ladies? I wonder if one of you might volunteer to describe your impressions as I signed to the deaf?'

After a few seconds during which no one responded to his request, a slight, middle-aged woman raised a gloved hand and Robert bade her speak while he signed her meaning to the deaf people.

'It all looked very strange and intriguing, Mr Kinniburgh,' she began, 'but I was confused. I didn't know what you were saying to them.'

There were murmurs of agreement throughout the congregation.

'Madam,' asked Robert, 'is it safe to say that you felt left out, in ignorance of what was going on?'

The woman nodded. 'I suppose I did.'

'And for how long would you estimate that the entire exchange of signs lasted?'

She shrugged. 'Ten minutes, perhaps?'

'Nothing like as long as that, madam' – Robert's face was serious now – 'less than two minutes. You see, ladies and gentlemen, when I was signing to the deaf, this lady, like the rest of you, was shut out from our conversation. That sense of exclusion magnified her perception of the length of time that the exchange actually lasted for. When we are made to feel unwelcome, time drags extremely slowly.'

Robert repeated his introduction for the hearing people and then carried on, laying out his thinking as to the cause of much of the deaf's strife.

'You see, most of us here tonight have been bestowed with the gift of hearing. We can listen to so much: the gossip and chatter of our fellows; the praise or admonishment of teachers and employers; notes of the sweetest music or the tendernesses of our loved ones. Yet do we ever consider the value of this gift that we have been given? We do not. We take it utterly for granted. We are oblivious to our good fortune and, because we do not appreciate our own privileges, by extension, we do not appreciate the privations that the deaf are subjected to.'

Robert paused for a moment to take a sip of water from his glass.

'What do I mean by privation? The deaf are treated unkindly in this world. Firstly, they are either born without the ability to hear or they lose that ability through accident or illness in infancy. Secondly, because they do not speak at all or they speak in a manner deemed unintelligible and unattractive to others, they are supposed to be ignorant and stupid. Thirdly, they are denied access to education and advancement because society can see no benefit to be procured from them and thus refuses to invest in their prospects.'

Robert indicated to David that he wished the young man to join him at the front of the church.

'I have lectured you for long enough. Instead of telling you how the deaf communicate, I would like to show you. I'm sure a few of you already know David Buchanan. To those who don't, let me introduce the son of our good reverend here.'

David smiled awkwardly at the assembly.

'I met David for the first time only last week,' explained Robert. 'Even at that first meeting we were able to communicate with each other using a combination of signs and finger-spelling. Some of our signs differed but many were the same. David has agreed to help me demonstrate sign language to you.'

Robert asked David his name and the young man replied, using his fingers to spell it out.

'This is a very basic exchange,' explained Robert, 'but it demonstrates perfectly the two complementary modes of this remarkable language: signs and the manual alphabet. I signed a question to David, and he spelled his answer out on his fingers. Let us look first at how deaf people manage the English alphabet.'

Robert asked David to spell his name again, slowly, for the benefit of the audience.

'So, you see,' said Robert, 'each shape is made by placing the right hand onto the left. The consonants are made by making shapes that correspond to the written letters. For example, the letter D is formed by curving the index finger and thumb of the right hand and joining it to the upright index finger of the left hand.' He finger-spelled it again to clarify. 'Whereas the letter V is made by placing the index and middle finger of the right hand, splayed onto the palm of the left hand. Like this.' Robert made the shape for V and raised it over his head so that everyone could see what he was doing.

'The other important aspect of our manual alphabet is that the vowels are demonstrated slightly differently,' Robert continued. 'The five fingers on the left hand are pointed at by the index finger of the right hand.'

Robert asked David to spell his name again.

'As you can see, the second letter of David's name is

an A, so he points to his thumb, whereas he points to his middle finger to indicate an I, the fourth letter of his Christian name.

'Simple and effective, is it not? But what if I wanted to tell David a story or give him directions or instructions? If I had to spell each letter out, it would take an incredibly long time. He would fall asleep with boredom before I reached the end. Imagine, for a moment, if you had to say each letter separately rather than running them together to make words and sentences that flow naturally from your mouth. It would be frustrating. If the deaf had to finger-spell everything that they wished to say – even if all were literate and had their alphabet – it would be an extremely ineffective mode of communication.'

Robert asked David to join him again.

'The solution is to make signs as an alternative to English words and phrases. It is not the same as speech. Instead, it is a visual and spatial movement better adapted to the needs of deaf people. Let me show you an example. Let us pretend that I have just met David in the street, and I am asking him about his destination.'

Robert turned to David. They greeted each other. *Hello. Where are you going?* Robert asked.

I'm going to church, answered David.

Where is your church?

It is in the East End, said David. *Almost a mile away.*

Robert asked the audience where they thought David was going to, if they had spotted any clues.

A man called out, 'He clasped his hands together. Was he going to pray?'

'Yes,' Robert said, demonstrating the sign, 'that's right. This is the sign for a church as well as for a prayer itself.'

Another man asked, 'When you asked him his destination,

you moved your hands as if you were proffering something in front of you. What did that mean?'

'This?' Robert held both his hands out in front of him, palms upwards. He moved his hands in circles as if he was polishing the bottom of a heavy saucepan. 'This is the sign for *where*?'

Those present were emboldened now. These initial questions had opened the floodgates and given them permission to be curious.

'Why did he gesture to the right?' asked a woman at the back of the hall.

Robert repeated the sign by pushing his straightened hand towards the right. 'This is how David indicated that he was travelling to the Calton, to the east of the city. If you can conceive of the signing area as a box in front of the body, we use that space to describe concepts and relationships. It is like a miniature stage where life is played out and situations explained. Deaf people communicate using a kinetic, three-dimensional language as opposed to our own linear, two-dimensional one.'

A young chap raised his hand. 'Mr Kinniburgh, who decides which signs are the correct ones to use?'

'That is an extremely good question, but the answer is somewhat complicated. There have always been deaf people and they have always attempted to find ways to communicate both with each other and with society in general. A number of examples have been recorded, stretching back centuries. The world has developed and become easier to navigate, and so communities of deaf people have shared their languages and a consensus of sorts has gradually developed. However, there are still huge differences, for example between the signs used in the Americas and in Great Britain. Also, where countries use different alphabets, it is almost impossible to follow what those deaf people are finger-spelling. However, the idea of signing seems to be common to all the groups of deaf people who have been studied so far.'

A young woman in a dark bonnet and heavy felt coat asked, 'Does a standard exist, whereby one can learn this language?'

Robert shook his head. 'Not as yet. There is no comprehensive or definitive guide to the signs used by deaf people. A standard alphabet for finger-spelling was published some years ago and there have been useful attempts to gather and illustrate a few of the most common signs.'

Robert looked around the room. 'Perhaps it would be instructive if I acted as interpreter and helped one of you converse with David?' he suggested.

The audience fell silent.

Robert laughed, 'Is anyone brave enough to volunteer?'

He pointed at the young woman who had asked the previous question. 'Miss, can I prevail upon you to help show these good people how simple it is?'

The young woman looked unsure but, egged on by her companions and encouraged by the crowd, she was induced to join Robert and David at the front of the room.

'Let us get to know each other,' said Robert. He pointed to David and pinched his hands together to indicate that he should start.

David waved his index finger and curled it, along with his middle finger, away from his forehead.

The young woman coloured and looked to Robert for guidance.

'What is your name?' Robert asked.

The young woman answered, 'Caroline Nimmo.'

Robert finger-spelled her name to David. Caroline followed his movements, biting her lip in concentration.

David made a sign by pointing his middle finger inward

and wiggling the others around. It was followed by the *where* sign that Robert had already explained.

'Where do you live?' Robert asked Caroline.

'I live in Weaver Street, off Rottenrow,' she answered.

Robert made the sign for street, two fingers of each hand running in front of him. And a sign for a weaver that mimicked a shuttle being drawn across a loom and the push of yarn into the waiting fabric.

David nodded as if he understood.

Robert looked enquiringly at David. He was not well acquainted with the topography of the city. How to sign Rottenrow?

In the end, Robert took the more laborious route and finger-spelled the word.

David laughed and showed him how to sign it. He made a sign for whiskers and then the sign for a road or a street or a path.

Robert shook his head, uncomprehendingly. *Why?* When David shrugged, Robert turned to the audience and asked them to explain why David would sign whiskers like a cat or a mouse to mean Rottenrow.

A tall man of patrician bearing, wearing an elaborate cravat in a dark-red paisley pattern, stood up. 'Rottenrow is a main road to the north of the city, Mr Kinniburgh,' he said. 'It is an ancient route and there is some debate over the meaning of its name. Some believe that is it derived from the Gaelic phrase *Rat-an-righ*, which translates loosely as the road of the kings – the idea being that royalty might use it to reach the cathedral. However, the name is common in towns and villages throughout the country where there once was a row of tumbledown cottages infested with rats, and so I think the whiskers the young man used might belong to those creatures.'

Robert thanked the man for this observation and

confessed himself fascinated with etymology. 'I hope we might talk later on the subject, sir? You seem quite the authority on the city.'

The wearer of the paisley cravat demurred but many in the audience agreed and Robert made a note to himself to seek this man out if he lingered after the lecture was over.

'To get back to our task in hand,' he continued. 'Now, Miss Nimmo, perhaps you would like to ask the same questions of David? First we will start with his name.' Robert demonstrated by asking David's name and then encouraged Caroline to copy what he had done, explaining the sequence in which she ought to do so. 'If you think about it in English, you are signing like this: Name? You? What? Would you like to try that with David?'

Caroline nodded and turned to the young man: *What is your name?*

David spelled the letters on his fingers.

Caroline turned back to Robert.

'To ask him where he lives, you do this,' he began, 'you can simply make the sign for *live* and the sign for *where* –' Robert demonstrated these signs once more – 'You don't have to sign *you* again because, if you are having a conversation and asking these kinds of questions, you both know who you are talking about.'

Caroline followed Robert's instructions and made the signs. David answered, *I live here, in the Calton, next to the church.*

At this, Caroline copied the new sign of *next* by jerking her thumb in the same manner as David and pointing to the right side of the church.

David laughed. With his hands an inch apart, he moved them as if rolling dough to make a small bread roll. *You know how to sign now.*

Caroline made the sign for *Thank you*. She flattened her hand with her fingertips on her chin and moved it outwards.

David placed both of his hands in a similar fashion and brought them forward, *You're welcome*.

Caroline watched him, rapt. She hadn't learnt the sign and yet she understood him.

Robert had hung back, letting them communicate directly with each other. The audience began to applaud enthusiastically. The tension in the room had dissipated. To hear them congratulate her, you would have thought that Miss Nimmo had acted in a Shakespearean tour-de-force rather than simply had a short conversation. Still, thought Robert, it was gratifying to be able to shift their mindset just a fraction.

~

When the lecture ended, some people left immediately. It was almost ten o'clock and many of them had travelled from outlying districts and needed to journey back to their homes by coach or on foot. Outside, it had turned bitterly cold, the day's sunshine too weak and short-lived to warm up the city streets for any length of time.

Those who remained milled about the church as Mr and Mrs Buchanan made enquiries of them and introduced them to others. Some of the younger deaf people busied themselves pouring drinks for the visitors and circulating with trays full of squares of sugary tablet. The women gravitated to one side of the church, clustered around Mrs Buchanan, the men to the open area in front of the pews.

Robert found himself in the midst of a crowd of well-to-do men, all firing questions at him that he struggled to answer before the next one struck him.

Eventually, the Reverend Buchanan interjected.

197

'I'm sure we would all like to hear of your work in the school, Mr Kinniburgh. Can you give us some idea of a typical lesson?'

'Certainly,' said Robert. 'My methods are more or less the same, regardless of what subject the class is studying. When the children begin at the school, we try to teach them their letters in order that they can garner information from books and learn in much the same way that hearing children do. However, we are always mindful that English is not their natural language, and it is not an ability that comes easily to them. Hearing children pick up language by listening to those around them. Deaf children do not. Their minds are just as curious and enquiring and so they find or make up alternative ways to communicate and that results in signing. For these reasons, I believe it is important to both encourage signing and English amongst the deaf.'

'What can we do to help you in this endeavour?' asked Angus.

'Well,' said Robert, 'there are two things, at the moment, that the institution needs: funds and pupils. Money can be pledged, in a variety of sums, either by subscribing to our pamphlet or by an individual donation. This money, as well as funding from their home parish, allows pupils to be sent to Edinburgh for an education. Thus, the opportunity to gain knowledge and skills and become a useful member of society is open not only to those born to wealthy families.'

'Do you think the time might come when Glasgow will have a school for the deaf and dumb of the same quality as your own institution?' Angus asked.

'I don't see why not,' Robert said. 'You are already doing good work here, the deaf are meeting and organising and their needs and desires are becoming more visible.

Perhaps by sending your deaf children to Edinburgh, we can educate them to be teachers and come back and establish a similar institution for the good of Glasgow.'

The crowd concurred. One man said, 'Anything Edinburgh can do, Glasgow can do, Mr Kinniburgh.'

Another man joined in. 'Anything Edinburgh can do, Glasgow can do better!'

This last was met with roars of approval.

Robert decided to press home his advantage.

'Gentlemen. Perhaps I can interest you in buying a copy of our annual pamphlet? I have some copies with me.'

Robert was soon surrounded by interested parties, gentlemen and their wives who wished to read more about his work. Every one of the little pamphlets, so ably illustrated by Margaret, were snapped up and Robert had to jot down the names and addresses of those who were disappointed and promise to send a copy on to them as soon as he returned to Edinburgh.

The man in the paisley-patterned cravat, who had been so knowledgeable about Rottenrow, asked to be added to his list.

'My name is Edward Ross, Mr Kinniburgh, I am also a teacher. At a boys' school on Argyle Street. I would be so grateful to read more about your school and share it with my pupils.'

'That would be wonderful,' replied Robert. 'The more the young can learn about the deaf, the easier it will be in the future for communication between everyone.'

'I must admit,' Ross continued, 'I was rather struck by the noises and the facial expressions of the deaf.'

Another man, who had been listening, interjected, 'Alarming, weren't they? I thought them exaggerated and slightly comical. Could be a bit threatening if you met a group of them on a dark night!'

The man chuckled, pleased at his joke, and Robert bristled. 'I suppose that may be true, if you think of the deaf as *other*, not like yourself.'

The man looked at Robert incredulously, 'Well, they *are* different from us, surely you can't deny that, Mr Kinniburgh?'

'I'm very much afraid that I can. The precise mode of communication might be different but the essence of it is exactly the same. I'm sorry, Mr . . . I don't believe we've been introduced?'

'My name is Charles McDougall.' The man proffered his hand and Robert shook it.

McDougall cast his eyes around the room and then fixed Robert with an appraising gaze. 'I suppose for those of a romantic bent, they have something of the noble savage about them. The deaf, that is. I don't see it myself.'

Robert said nothing.

McDougall continued, 'Some of them have found useful employment. We have people like the Reverend Buchanan to thank for that. I'm afraid that, in my experience, I've never found them to be satisfactory employees.'

The man was obviously waiting for a rejoinder and Robert reluctantly gave in.

'Really?' he asked. 'Why is that, do you think, Mr McDougall?'

McDougall inhaled deeply. Readying himself to deliver a lecture, Robert thought, defeatedly.

'They have few discernible skills to offer and, even when given a chance, make no attempt to get along with others. I took a couple of deaf and dumb lads on last year, to help with loading and unloading at the docks, but both of them took no instruction and were a liability to the business. After a week of spillages and accidents, I had to let them go.'

Robert said, 'It can be difficult to convey instructions

to a deaf person. Especially if you have not had prior experience of them or lack the time to invest to set them off on the right track. It can take longer to train the deaf but that is usually due to the difficulties in communication rather than a defect originating from the deafness itself.'

'Perhaps,' said McDougall. 'I am sure you have more insight into the needs of these unfortunates than I do, Mr Kinniburgh. I admit that I have little patience with those who are less quick-witted than I am. It is a failing of mine to expect the same of others as I do of myself.'

McDougall had a copy of Robert's pamphlet in his hand. Robert was sure he hadn't spoken to him earlier or made a note of his name. Perhaps another gentleman had given it to him to peruse. McDougall flicked through the pages until he came to a list of names.

'These are your patrons, I see?'

'Yes,' Robert answered, unsure of where this was going.

'I know this fellow,' McDougall said, pointing at the list of names, 'Andrew Carmichael. I've done business with him in the past.'

'Yes, Mr Carmichael has been one of our patrons since my predecessor was in post. He is always very generous with his time.'

'And his money, no doubt.' Again, the self-regarding chuckle.

'That goes without saying,' Robert replied.

'Do you give these talks often, Mr Kinniburgh?'

'As often as my duties at the school allow,' Robert replied. 'It is useful to travel outwith the capital and spread the word about what we are doing. Many families with deaf children are not aware that our provision exists, and parish councils are generally at a loss as to how to educate the deaf children they have responsibility for.'

'But your teaching is confined to Edinburgh, is that right?'

'Yes. At least for the moment. Some of the older children in my care are undertaking some teaching duties with younger pupils and, as time goes on, I hope to enlist their assistance in training hearing teachers to instruct deaf pupils elsewhere in the country. Along the lines of the model we have developed at the institution.'

McDougall looked surprised. 'Remarkable. Do you think it worth the effort, Mr Kinniburgh, to promote the deaf to a higher level of education? Surely they are capable only of manual work of some kind?'

'Not at all, Mr McDougall,' said Robert, incredulously. 'They are capable of the same achievements as hearing people are.'

McDougall smiled. As if he knew better.

Robert decided to change the subject. 'And how are you connected with the reverend's church, Mr McDougall?' he asked.

McDougall affected to be deep in thought about this question. Trying to give the impression it was hard to untangle his copious commitments, Robert suspected. 'I sit on the Benevolent Fund Committee at the Merchants' Hall. It's important that commerce, which does so well in our burgeoning city, is seen to salve the wounds of those who are suffering, don't you agree?'

Robert's head dipped, begrudgingly. He had taken against this man from the outset, regarding his comments about deaf people as ignorant and distasteful. In addition, Mr McDougall had a self-righteous air about him. Robert tried not to judge; sometimes it was difficult, but he knew he really ought to leave that to God.

'And you, Mr Kinniburgh?' said McDougall. 'What made you choose to visit Reverend Buchanan's small church in the Calton? I'm sure there must be more lucrative avenues for you to explore in our metropolis.'

'I was here on business that caused me to cross paths with the reverend,' said Robert.

'Indeed? What business was that?' McDougall asked.

'I have been appointed by the courts to assist in the case of the unfortunate deaf lady lately taken from Glasgow and awaiting trial on a charge of murder. I have been trying to speak to some of those she was in contact with immediately before the incident.'

'Really?' McDougall said, raising an eyebrow in an almost pantomime fashion.

Robert realised he had let his vanity get the better of him. He immediately regretted sharing this information with McDougall.

There was a pause as McDougall waited for Robert to carry on. When the silence remained, he decided to fill it himself.

'This is the case of the baby that was thrown from the Old Bridge?'

Robert nodded.

'And is she to be put on trial for murder, Mr Kinniburgh?'

Robert shrugged. 'That will be up to the judiciary to decide. Lord Succoth has been tasked with determining her fitness to plead. At the moment I am simply trying to make sense of her story in order to relay it to His Lordship.'

'And that has led you to Glasgow?' McDougall asked.

'Yes.'

'And have you found those that you came to seek out?'

'Some of them, yes,' Robert said. 'I am still attempting to find the whereabouts of her common-law husband.'

'You think the fellow has something to do with the baby's death?'

Robert hesitated.

'I have heard some whispers about the Irishman,' said McDougall.

'Really?' said Robert.

'The talk is all about the fact that the man, I forget his name . . .'

'Donnelly,' said Robert. 'James Donnelly is his name.'

McDougall smiled. 'Ah, yes. The talk is that this Donnelly is wanted by the authorities back in his home country. For what I have no idea, but it wouldn't surprise me in the least. They are a rough crowd, the Irishmen who make their way to our city.'

'Where did you hear this?' Robert asked.

'My labourers talk amongst themselves,' McDougall said. 'I don't employ papists myself but the men who work for me hear these rumours down at the docks. The information reached my ears by some circuitous route, no doubt, I don't quite recall. Normally, I set little store by these stories but, in this case . . .' McDougall made a show of ruminating on the gossip he had just imparted.

'I have left a message for the Donnelly fellow at his lodgings,' said Robert. 'Hopefully I will be able to catch up with him and make my own judgement about him.'

'I imagine he'll be long gone by now,' said McDougall. 'And, if by some small chance he's still in Glasgow and he receives your message, he's more likely to take it as a warning rather than an invitation.'

'Perhaps,' Robert said.

McDougall was momentarily distracted by another man who called over to him to ask if he wished to share his carriage.

'Well, Mr Kinniburgh, I must away. I wish you every success in bringing the case to a speedy conclusion. I wouldn't worry too much, mind, if the man Donnelly can't be found. Even if the papist was involved, Campbell is surely guilty too.' McDougall continued, 'What was the woman thinking, Kinniburgh, running around the streets with her child's dead body?'

Robert was brought up short by this question. He stood for a minute, digesting McDougall's parting words. Nobody except himself and Jean knew that the baby was dead before it was lost to the river.

40

~ Wednesday, 12 March 1817:
Miller's Court, Glasgow ~

The jeweller's workshop was on the third floor of the building. The door was fitted with a heavy mortice lock. David Buchanan turned the key and let himself in.

It was still dark outside, although the birds had begun to sing. They perched on rooftops where weeds flourished in the cracks between slates. There were scant pickings here, but sparrows and coal tits had set up home, building nests out of the detritus from the skimble-scamble of shops and businesses that converged upon George Square.

A jumble of tools lay haphazardly on the counter and David began tidying them away, wiping each thoroughly with a rag and placing it in a huge set of drawers that lined the far wall. This storage system was made of an old oak cabinet and had been supplemented over the years with hastily made or adapted shelves and hooks to accommodate the tools of the trade as well as a huge variety of abandoned links, chain and clasps that were more than likely to come in handy in the future.

A smell of day-old blood and faeces crept up from the beef and mutton market at the corner of John Street. Even here, in the broad streets around the square, smells proliferated and trickled in through tiny gaps in closed windows. It was pervasive, this stench of animal. Beasts were herded to the city to be bought and sold and every piece of them was used. The carcasses taken to be tanned, meat jointed and jugged, hair and bones disseminated to a myriad of cottage industries that had need of them, and any leftovers scavenged by the poor and turned to some small advantage. The enterprise was so comprehensive that it left no visible trace; only the odour of the natural world after it had been stripped and processed.

David was still half asleep; it had been a monumental effort to rouse himself from his warm bed for this earliest of shifts. His employer, Gillespie, had sent by letter for him the previous evening and bade him come in early, as there was a long list of customers' orders waiting to be fulfilled. Gillespie had been poorly of late and much slower at his work. As a result, he relied more and more on David to take up the slack, not only to complete the work but to supervise a new apprentice into the bargain. Despite his weariness, David was glad to help out, grateful as he was to Mr Gillespie for giving him his start and training him up in the trade. He had the skill and concentration for close work and an amiability that allowed him to get on with people, despite not hearing what they said. Many of the jeweller's customers, who came regularly and often, were either private clients from the upper echelons of society who trusted Gillespie to repair their precious items, or shopkeepers who traded in gentlemen's watches or ladies' jewellery but who lacked the training to make their own repairs. These people had been introduced to David from the time he began his apprenticeship and were comfortable communicating with him using rudimentary signs or scribbling instructions and diagrams on pieces of paper. David had been schooled by his father and was able to read and write to a decent standard and had, in fact, more education than most of the hearing people that lived and worked in the city.

Gillespie's customers had got to know David over the

years and fully expected him to take over the business in due course. David himself was amenable to that idea, though he had never discussed it directly with his employer. Up until recently, it had seemed a long way off but, with Mr Gillespie so ill, David had begun to wonder about it. His employer had no son, only a daughter, and it was likely that David would be his chosen heir. However, should Gillespie's ill health continue and force him to sell the business, it was by no means guaranteed that a new owner would want to take David on as well.

He began to sweep the counter with a small dustpan and brush, coaxing out the tiny fragments of details and stones that had accumulated in every crevice.

The door to the workshop opened and he looked up. He was surprised to see Robert cross the threshold and close the door behind him.

Good morning, Robert signed.

David nodded a greeting in return.

Are you very busy? Robert asked. *I should like to speak with you.*

Busy, yes, David answered. *But, if you can wait until I finish clearing up, we can talk.*

I can give you a hand, if you like, Robert suggested.

When the workshop was straightened up, Robert told David about his quest. *I'm on my way to the Merchants' Hall. I'm looking for an address for a man, McDougall. I think it possible that he is the man who Jean talks about. Can you help me?*

David nodded. *What do you want me to do?*

Come with me to visit him when I find out where he lives?

David had no hesitation. *Of course. I can come with you. I'll need to finish my work here, but I could be ready this afternoon. About three o'clock?*

Robert nodded. *Yes. I can come back then.*

What do you mean to do when we get there? David asked.

Robert rolled his eyes. *I'm hoping to have formulated a plan when I return.*

～

The doors to the Merchants' Hall were locked and bolted when Robert rapped on them half an hour later. He had hoped that someone would be abroad by now. It was his understanding that, as well as the shops on the ground floor, the building was home to a small number of old and destitute merchants, the more able-bodied of whom helped out by undertaking various administrative and janitorial tasks.

It was still fairly early, he thought. Perhaps these old relics took a while to breakfast. No need to give up. He decided to take a wander around the area so that he could easily check if anyone had opened the hall.

He picked his way along a narrow vennel and found himself on an embankment that dropped down to the river. To the east, the Clyde narrowed on its approach to the Green but, to the west, the river was crowded on both sides by numerous quays – one or two well-built and substantial but some mere rickety structures cobbled together from random pieces of salvaged wood. The water was deeper here and lapped up the sides of the embankment.

Robert could see how easy it would be for the river to flood and overwhelm the buildings built so close to it. The Merchants' Hall was set back a little from the riverbank, but many buildings were nearer and were in the process of being taken down or had been abandoned to the elements. Glasgow was a city that had begun to reap rewards from the river, but it was also subject to its caprices.

Where the water was shallower on the north bank, Robert watched as figures moved slowly amidst the mud and silt underneath him. Shadows, whose habit was almost indistinguishable from their surroundings. Robert studied them as they intersected and then diverged from each other, each bending down periodically to lift something from the river, inspect it and then either tuck it away in their clothing or discard it, depending on its value. These people were looking for any scrap of bone or rope that could be sold for a pittance and exchanged, in turn, for bread or shelter for the night.

A boy called up at him from the riverbed. He had a shock of unruly brown hair that looked like it had been hacked at by a set of farming shears. His rolled trousers were held up courtesy of a pair of braces over a thin, bare chest. The boy stood, hands on hips, surveying Robert.

'Any spare coin, sir?'

Robert rummaged in his pocket and took out a few coins. He didn't want to throw them onto the wet bank, fearful that the mud might swallow them up before the boy could reach them. He hunkered down and passed them into the boy's outstretched hand.

'Much obliged, sir.' The boy nodded at Robert and returned to his scavenging.

When he had retraced his steps, Robert found that the Merchants' Hall had been opened. In the lobby, a woman who was sweeping the floor pointed him in the direction of a small window. When Robert knocked on the window it was opened by a bald man who listened to his request and furnished him with an address for Charles McDougall.

Partickhill Road. Robert had no idea where that was, but he thanked the man for his help, and hoped David would have an idea of how they might get there.

~

Later that afternoon, Robert and David walked to George Square with the intention of procuring a ride to Partick. The square was a jostle of pedestrians, horses, carts and coaches. Robert was inclined to look for a coach for hire, but David directed him towards the carters who were loading up for their trips out of the city.

Once aboard a cart piled with cases of provisions bound westwards, they both stretched out, planting their backs on one side and their feet on the other to give them some purchase as defence against the jolts of the journey.

When we get there, what will we do? David asked.

We'll ask for McDougall, Robert said. *I'll tell him that we're looking for people to speak up for Jean. Try to get inside. See how he reacts.*

David nodded and grinned as they hit a pothole and Robert's hat went flying across the cart, sending the schoolmaster scrabbling to retrieve it before it fell out.

They reached Partickhill within half an hour. Robert hailed a man who was walking on the other side of the road. 'Could you point us in the direction of the McDougall house?' he asked.

'Just up the brae, there,' the man indicated. 'You see the house with the slate roof and long stone wall?'

Robert did. He nodded his thanks and he and David carried on.

The house at Partickhill was in darkness. Robert knocked at the door, but he did so in the sure and certain knowledge that no one was at home. The blinds and curtains were drawn in every room. Both men walked around the house to the back door, which was also securely locked and bolted.

How strange, thought Robert, the man at the Merchants' Hall had told him that Charles McDougall lived at this villa with his wife and servants. Even if the McDougalls had left for a few days, surely a servant would be in attendance. And yet there was no one.

41

∼ Wednesday, 12 March 1817:
Partick, Glasgow ∼

The afternoon sun warmed them even as it began to dip westwards towards the river, but a restlessness settled on the two men. Since finding the McDougall house shut up, they had lost much of their previous focus and determination.

Stopping at the side of the road, Robert laid a hand on David's shoulder. *Should we go back into Glasgow?*

Yes, if you think there is nothing more to be done here?

We could make enquiries somewhere, said Robert, *but I wouldn't know where to start.*

David pointed down the hill. *There's bound to be an inn or a shop near the Clyde. Why don't we head towards those houses?*

As they retraced their steps towards the Dumbarton Road, the village proper began to materialise. They crossed over at a junction that led down to the river in the direction of Meadowside. Here, the Clyde was narrow and dotted with inches – raised beds of sand and silt that acted as islands. At this point in the river, only small boats might pass, so larger ships often offloaded cargo that was then carted into Glasgow. This was a hindrance to trade and the city fathers planned what had been termed a canalisation of this stretch of the Clyde, to widen and deepen the channel and allow larger boats to pass all the way to the centre of the city. This meant raising and strengthening the banks, changing natural slopes into proper quays and walls. Some preparations were already taking place, with trenches being dug and temporarily shored up with wooden planks.

A group of working men were sitting to the side of one of these endeavours, the sweat of toil still evident on their brows as they puffed away at pipes and drank out of hip flasks.

'Would you know a place we might get a drink and rest a while?' Robert asked them and they gestured in the direction of a small cottage close to the water. Robert and David followed the instruction and found themselves on the threshold of a chandler's that had a public bar with a few tables in the back of the shop. They ordered two small beers and settled down at a low table.

When the shopkeeper brought their drinks over, Robert asked him if he knew of an engineer by the name of McDougall.

The man rubbed his hands on his leather apron and nodded.

'I do. Runs a workshop around the corner and has a few boats on the river. He's involved with the improvement works too, I believe.'

'Aye,' said Robert, 'I'd heard that. My friend and I were wanting to speak to him but there's no one at his house further up the hill. Has anything been seen of him recently?'

'A couple of his men were in here a few days ago. I heard talk of McDougall sleeping at the workshop. The men said he was there in the mornings a couple of times; early doors when they turned up for work.'

'Why did they think he'd been sleeping there?' Robert asked.

The shopkeeper shrugged. 'He just looked crumpled, you know? Hadn't shaved and he looked like he'd slept in his clothes. His men assumed McDougall had been sleeping off a night on the tiles or maybe fallen out with the wife. Then he seemed to disappear for a few days and the word was the house was shut up.'

Robert turned to David and imparted the gist of this conversation to him. The deaf man looked curious.

Why is there no one there? David asked.

'Do you know why he shut up the house?' asked Robert.

'No really, sir. One of the local women stopped working for him, and a wee lassie that lived in, she's back at her mother and father's place now. They've not got much to say about it right enough.'

'Where would I find this woman and the girl?'

'I think they both stay on Castlebank Street, sir. No sure the exact houses, mind. If you go back the way you came and turn right, there's a stretch of dwellings. You'll likely find them there. The old woman's a Mrs Drysdale. I cannae mind the lassie's first name but her father's cried Sproull.'

Robert clapped David on the back and signed to him. *Two people who worked at the McDougall house live close by. Would you try to find them with me?*

David grinned. *Lead on.*

~

It was easy enough to find the cottages. Once they were on the right stretch of road, folk were more than happy to point them in the direction of the Drysdale and Sproull households.

The families lived only two doors apart in similar wooden and thatched buildings. Although the village of Partick was being assailed on all sides by the changes wrought by industry, the place was still dotted with small groups of houses that looked like they had been there since medieval times. Here, unlike in the ghettos in the eastern stretch of Glasgow, walls had been shored up and improvements made. Everything was neat and tidy, and people had space to wash and dry their clothing. Many kept livestock on the land opposite their houses and grew vegetables to feed their families and trade with neighbours for other necessities.

Robert rapped on the door of the Drysdales' cottage with no success. David peered through a small, grubby window but could see no sign of life.

At the Sproull girl's house, a middle-aged woman answered the door and Robert explained that he was looking for her daughter.

She looked at him askance. 'Which one of my daughters would you mean, sir?' The woman gave the distinct impression that she did not trust Robert's intentions.

'I'm afraid I don't know her name. She worked for the McDougalls in Partickhill.'

'That's our Martha,' the woman replied, before seeming to check herself. 'What do you want with her?'

'I'm endeavouring to get in touch with her employer, Mr McDougall,' Robert said. 'I need to ask him some questions about a woman called Jean Campbell. I'm a friend of hers, working on her behalf. Jean is to stand trial for murder, and I believe McDougall may have had something to do with the crime she is accused of.'

'Our Martha wouldn't know anything about that,' Mrs Sproull said, bluntly.

Robert faltered. 'I don't seek to implicate your daughter in anything, Mrs Sproull, please be assured of that. I only meant to ask her for her help in locating McDougall. Would it be possible to have a word with her?'

'She's at her work,' came the terse reply.

David, who had been standing patiently all this time, suddenly asked, *What's wrong? Is the girl here or not?*

Robert shook his head. *She's out at work.*

Mrs Sproull recoiled at David's interjection, treating both him and Robert with even more suspicion than before. She closed the door over, leaving the two men scratching their heads at what to do next. A moment later, however, the door opened again.

'You say you're a friend of the deaf woman, Jean?'

'I am, yes, Mrs Sproull,' said Robert. 'I am to help her give evidence to the jury. She told me that she was ill-treated by the McDougalls and has intimated that it was they, and not her, who killed her baby.'

Robert was surprised to see tears in Mrs Sproull's eyes and realised that her carapace was little more than a flimsy defence.

'Our Martha was right fond of the woman. It's terrible what happened to her child.'

'Might your daughter know something that could assist me?' asked Robert. 'Jean tells me the baby was killed inside the house, not by drowning at the Old Bridge, as is alleged.'

Mrs Sproull smoothed her apron and thought for a moment. 'Martha doesn't know how the baby died. She was sent downstairs and the next thing she knew was that Jean had ran away. There's no point asking her questions, that's all she knows, and she won't be drawn on McDougall. She doesn't trust him one little bit.'

'You say yourself that your daughter cared about Jean. Surely she would be willing to help her?'

'What can Martha tell you that would help Jean? I've told you she didn't see anything. She's better keeping away from the McDougalls altogether. That's what she wants and her father and me agree.'

Robert reached inside his jacket pocket and pulled out a silver case. 'Would you take my card, regardless?'

'She'll not change her mind,' Mrs Sproull sighed, taking

the card anyway, and Robert had to concede that she was probably right.

'And Mrs Drysdale, who was cook at the McDougall house, have you any idea where she is now?'

'Gone this last week,' said Mrs Sproull. 'Her and her man have given up their lodgings and gone to live with her sister, somewhere near the coast. Her man's bad with his chest so he is. They're hoping the sea air will do him some good.'

'Would you know where that might be?' Robert asked.

Mrs Sproull shook her head.

Robert covered his eyes with his hand. He thought he might weep with frustration. It was as if he had been watching a play where the curtain had arisen on the final act, only to reveal most of the main players and supporting cast inexplicably killed off. McDougall and his wife appeared to be long gone and anyone who could shed light on what had happened at their villa had either vanished or was too frightened to open their mouths in support of Jean. He couldn't blame Martha, dispiriting though it was to accept her reticence.

He stood up and looked dejectedly at David. *There is nothing more to be done here. No one to back up Jean's account. We should go.*

Robert and David nodded their thanks but, just as Mrs Sproull made to close her door, a girl approached them on the narrow road. She looked confusedly at Mrs Sproull's anxious expression and Robert suddenly understood.

'Martha?'

The girl stopped in her tracks and looked at him. Robert thought he could see fear in her eyes.

'My name is Robert Kinniburgh. I'm a teacher of the deaf. I need you to help me. I need to prove Jean Campbell's not a murderess.'

Martha's eyes widened. 'She's not. She'd never have harmed her wee boy. She only wanted the best for Donnie.'

Robert gasped. Until now the victim of this crime had been at worst a missing corpse, at best an unchristened baby, a soul denied salvation. It shocked him to the core that he had never stopped to consider whether Jean's baby had been given a name.

Robert stepped to one side to give the girl room. 'Did you see who killed Jean's son, Martha?'

Martha shook her head. 'The mistress was angry, at me, at Jean, I think at the baby too. The baby was crying and she took it away to her bedroom. The master arrived and Mrs Drysdale, the cook, brought me downstairs. I heard Jean screaming and then there was silence for a few minutes. The next thing I heard was the front door slam and Jean and the baby were gone.'

'What do you think happened?' asked Robert.

'I don't know, sir. I'm sorry but I just don't know for sure. Why would Jean kill her own baby?'

'What about Mrs McDougall?' Robert asked. 'You said she was angry. Could she have been angry enough to hurt a child?'

'She's a very unhappy woman. There was no love in the house, but I thought the baby might've made things better.'

'Perhaps the arrival of the poor child made things worse?'

Martha nodded. 'The mistress hated Jean, even before the baby arrived,' she said. 'She wouldn't look at her. Kept to her room. She started hurting herself too.'

'What do you mean, hurting herself?' Robert asked.

'She would cut her skin and let it bleed. Dr Wilson was often in the house. With dressings and such. I would find the master's razor lying, so I'd wipe it and put it away.'

The girl cast her eyes downwards. As if she were

ashamed of collusion. Robert felt a rush of sympathy for this girl, little more than a child really, who must have felt bewildered and alone in the midst of the McDougalls' bitter union.

'You did right, Martha,' Robert said. 'You looked after your mistress the best you could. The things that happened in that house were not your responsibility.'

Martha considered this for a moment. 'I don't think the mistress wanted a baby. Not even if it had been her own child. I know that's an unnatural thing for a woman, but it was Mr McDougall that wanted a child and everything he did made the mistress suffer.'

'It is every husband's duty. The Lord exhorts us to go forth and multiply,' said Robert. 'He was only doing God's will.'

Martha shrugged. 'I know my Bible, sir, and all I can say is that our Lord's word isn't always used in a Christian way. Not in that house, at any rate.'

Robert cast his eyes downwards. His instinct ought to have been to argue against Martha's position, but he was no longer completely sure of his own.

'Do you have any idea where Mrs McDougall is now?'

'Dr Wilson told me she was to go to some kind of hospital, sir. He had me pack a deal of her things into a trunk and he came to collect her in a private coach.'

'He didn't say which hospital?'

'No. But I heard the master muttering about her being a lunatic, so I wondered if it was some kind of asylum she was bound for.'

'I see.'

'Where is Jean, sir? Is she alright?'

'She's in Edinburgh, awaiting trial. She's well enough, but if I can't prove that someone else killed her son, she'll be hanged for murder.'

Martha began to cry. 'I'm heart sorry for her, so I am.' She thrust her hands into the front pocket of her apron and brought out a piece of ribboned cotton. 'I kept this. It's the cap the baby was wearing that day. Would you give it to Jean for me?'

Robert looked at the tiny piece of material she held in her outstretched palm.

'Of course I will, Martha. Thank you. I feel sure it will give her some comfort.'

~

Martha watched as the two men turned the corner to take them back to the main road and pushed back the memories that threatened to spill into her consciousness. There was too much she couldn't make sense of.

She was not simply frightened to recall the violence that occurred in the McDougalls' house – she remembered more about that day than simply the act that shattered it. She had proved unable to reconcile herself to the contrast between how the day began and how it ended.

Martha could barely visualise the reality of the dead baby. Despite the horror of what happened, the abiding memory she had of that day was of a baby who breathed and fed and cried and cleaved to his mother.

Who needed her even when he stopped doing all of those things. When he was stopped from doing those things.

42

∼ Monday, 24 February 1817:
Partickhill Road, Glasgow ∼

They were in the nursery; Martha, Jean and the baby. Jean had fed him, and Martha had changed him, and they had lain him down on the bed. Martha was tickling him on the soles of his feet. Jean was folding his used napkin into a bucket by the side of the bed with a wooden paddle that was suspended in cold water.

The bucket had a lid on it to make it easier to transport downstairs for laundering. Martha still had that job to do, but she was in no hurry to move from the nursery, since the fire was burning there.

Jean had made it plain that she welcomed her company. They got on well together. That Martha clearly didn't think much to the pair of them, her master and mistress, only seemed to commend her more in Jean's view.

Martha had told Jean that Ina felt sorry for the mistress, but all the sympathy Martha had known had been squandered. Earlier that day, the bell had rung in the kitchen, summoning Martha to the front room. When she arrived, the master and mistress were sitting in armchairs facing one another, she holding the shawl-wrapped bundle and he concealed behind a newspaper. Martha was sure she had seen the mistress nip the baby, and she suspected this had been done as an excuse to offload him.

'Baby's needing changed,' Mrs McDougall said as the wee soul whimpered. The mistress held the baby out in front of her, grudgingly cupping his head, as if waiting for Martha to relieve her of an intolerable burden.

Martha had brought him upstairs. When the baby was in Jean's arms, he cooried into her breast, and it was obvious that all he'd wanted was a feed. They'd changed him afterwards anyway. Martha put more coal on the fire – taking her time while Jean laid out clean clothes on the counterpane, his vest and blouson, his knitted hose, snug jerkin and ribboned bonnet. She and Martha made a game of it. Jean kissed all of his fingers and all of his toes. Martha, meanwhile, sang a song that she remembered from her own childhood.

They had forgotten all about the mistress and so were caught completely off guard when she appeared in the doorway to the nursery. She had evidently come directly from her bedroom, because her gown was unbuttoned, and her hair dishevelled. Her skin looked clammy, almost waxen, and Martha wondered if she had taken some of Dr Wilson's powders. Martha thought that she looked like a malevolent phantom from the pages of a storybook.

Martha and Jean stared at each other for a second, unsure at how to react to this visitor. They did not know what they had done wrong, but they were under no illusion that there must be something.

It was as if their pleasure in spending a little time in comforting the baby, making him the centre of their attention for once instead of the cause of their endless chores, had somehow overbalanced the scales in the house at Partickhill.

'Can't you stop this infernal racket?' snapped Mrs McDougall.

Jean regarded her as she might a snarling dog that had cornered her in a tight spot.

'We're just changing the baby, madam,' Martha said, but

the mistress was not listening. She was watching Jean intently.

Jean, for her part, stared calmly back at her, unmoving, not giving any ground.

Mrs McDougall turned to Martha. 'Get out.'

Martha stood up and glanced back at the deaf woman apologetically, but there was no need. Jean shook her head as if to say, *Don't worry, it's not your fault.*

Martha moved towards the door.

'Take this mess with you, you stupid girl.'

Martha baulked but grabbed the handle of the pail.

She'd had enough of this nasty boot. She was paid help, not a slave to order about. On her next day off, she'd go straight home and tell her father about this woman. He'd find her another place, somewhere she wouldn't get treated like this. Once she told him what the McDougalls were like, he wouldn't let her come back, wage or no wage.

In her haste to get out of the room, Martha stumbled, and the pail banged against the side of the bed, spilling some of its contents on to the floor.

Mrs McDougall's fury erupted and, weak as she was, her arm shot out from her side and delivered a stinging blow to the side of Martha's face, the jagged settings of her engagement ring catching the taut skin near the girl's eye. As Martha stared at her mistress in disbelief, Jean sped across the room and slapped Mrs McDougall hard across her jaw, knocking her almost to the floor.

Yet the mistress rallied. She snatched up the baby and ran out of the door, along the hallway and into her bedroom, leaving Jean and Martha staring incredulously at one another.

43

*~ Monday, 24 February 1817:
Partickhill Road, Glasgow ~*

Euphemia leant hard against the bedroom door. With her free hand, she reached down and turned the key in the lock. The metal was cold against her fingertips. She was clutching the baby so tightly that his cries were muffled now, all of his hurt concentrated in the heaving motion of his chest against hers.

And yet, the baby seemed anything but helpless in Euphemia's mind. It was monstrous and all-pervasive. Where others saw a cherub, a treasure, she saw only a demon who got bigger and fatter each day with every ounce of his mother's milk.

She heard footsteps flying along the upstairs landing and Jean began to pound on the door. She was screaming; a mixture of grunts and whelps and half-formed words spewing forth.

Euphemia rolled her eyes. She had no idea why people described these creatures as *mute* – this one never stopped with her racket. Euphemia's stomach turned. The deaf woman was like something that had crawled out from a primeval swamp. An illiterate bitch with nothing better to do than produce children. She ought to be grateful to be given the chance to elevate her lumpen offspring into a class far above her own. On the contrary, thought Euphemia, she has no imagination or ambition, cannot appreciate the opportunity bestowed upon her.

Euphemia suddenly became aware of the infant imprisoned in her grasp and recoiled, holding it out at arm's length, well away from her body. The smell of it made her gag. It had cried so hard and so long that her dress was sticky with snot.

This child was less than nothing to her. A mewling, piss-stained, shitting lump of flesh. The product of an idiot hoor and a dirty taig. What had possessed Charles that he should have expected her to care for it? Even a woman of her class, with servants to feed and clothe it and clean its mess up, was still required to hold the infant or to gaze adoringly at it, swaddled in its crib. Had Charles thought for a single instant that would be a task that she would find remotely achievable?

Such a stupid man. Arrogant and possessed of a belief that money can buy anything. She had never wanted a baby. It was Charles who wanted that, who had a list of checks and balances in an imaginary ledger marked *Home*. He had earned a place in society and married judiciously. Now he must have a child to reflect his status and show the world the extent of his virility.

~

Euphemia could hear Charles now. He was outside the door. He was shouting her name, telling her to open the door this minute, stop this shameful behaviour. The words were prescriptive, demanding, but there was rising panic in the tone of his voice.

The baby had quietened a little but, when she put it down on the bed, it began to mewl again. Ignorant, selfish creature; couldn't it see that these noises hurt her? Why couldn't she be left in peace?

Charles was banging on the door now, shouting

226

obscenities, threatening violence. Why did he think that would induce her to open the door to him?

She crouched on the floor, squeezing herself into the tiniest space she could, knowing all the time that there was nowhere to escape to. No place where she could be alone or catch her breath for an instant.

The baby began to howl again.

She dragged herself up to a standing position and picked it up, tried to hold it close, but it repulsed her. She began jiggling it around but that only increased its cries.

What she needed to do was to shut the thing up.

Euphemia threw the baby to the ground and an almighty crack reverberated around the room.

The noise stopped.

A leggy spider, dislodged from a dark corner of the fireplace, moved skittishly across the skating-rink surface of the hearthstone.

Euphemia watched its progress, wondering what would happen if its thread-like legs got caught up in the spreading liquid.

And the hoor outside in the hall, still rattling at the doorknob and wailing. She had no idea that silence had descended.

44

~ Monday, 24 February 1817:
Partickhill Road, Glasgow ~

An irregular trail of red spots dripped all the way to the upstairs landing. On the stone flags in the kitchen the spots pooled and hardened. On the carpeted stairs, they soaked into the patterned wool.

Martha plunged her arms into the scalding water. The scullery sink was filled with sheets from the mistress's bedroom and articles of her clothing. The water was soapy and dark with blood.

Martha had tried her hardest to contain the mess, but the magnitude of the task was beyond her. She'd cleaned up the mistress as best she could and bundled up the linen to take downstairs as the doctor had instructed. While that steeped in cold water, she'd began boiling more on the stove using the kettle and a soup pot, poured it in the sink when it was ready and set to boiling some more as she scrubbed. She went outside to the pump and filled up two more basins with cold water. She carried these inside and transferred the clothes and bedding, rinsed them and, dismayed with the results, began the process all over again.

Martha realised that her knees were shaking. It was almost comical, the force at which they were moving, completely out of her control. It reminded her of the time a gang of them had been playing near the river and she had been persuaded to climb on a rope swing suspended from a tree over the water. She was the youngest of the group by at least two years and had been dragged along by her older sister, Katie. Martha remembered that the terror of it, and the relief when it was over, all seemed to concentrate in her legs.

She focused on the washing and her knees dealt with the confusion for now. Martha couldn't do anything else to help. The doctor would look after the mistress. The master had gone out, where to she didn't know.

The mistress had taken the baby from Jean and locked her bedroom door and Jean had screamed and howled and battered her fists against it. She had watched as the master raced up the stairs towards his wife's room. Martha had made to follow him, but Ina had come to the lobby and the cook moved faster than Martha would have suspected a woman of her age was capable of. Ina had grabbed her by the arm and taken the pail with the dirty nappy from her. Martha had let herself be ushered downstairs to the kitchen like a sleepwalker guided back to the safety of her own bed.

Martha had just stood there. She couldn't make sense of how this had happened. Of what, in fact, had happened. A few minutes before, Jean had finished feeding the baby and she and Martha were changing his clothes, the wee soul lying on the bed kicking his legs. Martha and Jean laughing. A fire was burning in the grate, the small room was bright and cosy, and the wee boy was so beautiful.

Martha looked down at her hands, still rubbing and squeezing at the bloody stains on the mistress's clothing, working away almost instinctively. Mrs McDougall's chemise was soaked through, a surprising gradation in colour from the saturated cuffs to the splattered bodice; ruby and scarlet and crimson.

Martha came from a large family who lived in two rooms and a kitchen. She had helped as babies were born and washed out countless monthly rags for her mother and sisters. In her young life she had seen a lot of blood, but this was different. This was brought forth from somewhere unnatural, somewhere Martha didn't want to go.

Under the water, her fingers looked white. Her short housemaid's nails already old before their time. A lifetime of other people's laundry waiting for her.

45

~ Wednesday, 12 March 1817:
Calton, Glasgow ~

It was eight in the evening before Robert and David returned to the church. It being mild and dry, they had walked along the river from Partick, stopping only once to drink water from a well. Now they sat in the parlour of the manse with Angus. Mrs Buchanan had brought some oatcakes and ham and cheese but despite his hunger, Robert had little enthusiasm for eating.

'Must you go back to Edinburgh tomorrow, Robert?' asked Angus. 'Could you not stay another day or two? Given more time we might find McDougall.'

'Perhaps, but in all honesty, Angus, I can't see what that would be likely to achieve.'

'Don't lay down to defeatism, man,' Angus said. 'If you can find McDougall, he can be taken to task for his actions.'

Robert stretched, rolled his shoulders to ease the tension that he felt there.

'I know you mean well,' he said, 'but that is not the case. There is no evidence that either McDougall or his wife murdered Jean's baby. Even if the maid, Martha Sproull, was to testify, she can only place them upstairs at the time of the murder. They could easily blame each other or blame Jean and, if McDougall did attack Jean or the child near the bridge, there are no witnesses to corroborate it. Jean herself maintains the baby was dead by then. McDougall might be a liar and a brute, but I can't be sure that he's our murderer.'

'You must have faith,' Angus said. 'If Jean is innocent, then God hears her prayers and will take care of her.'

Robert sighed. 'I know God will look after her, I'd just prefer it to be when she's alive rather than dead.'

David looked up from his plate. *What are you two talking about?* he asked, pointing with his index fingers and banging his fists together.

Robert explained the situation to him. *How to help Jean when there is no proof that someone else killed her baby. I am worried. The events at the house in Partickhill are so bizarre that I am afraid the court will think her mad if she tries to explain them.*

And if they believe her to be mad, she will be locked away forever? David motioned a key turning and then signified the concept of *forever* by circling his index fingers around each other.

Robert nodded.

Which is worse? David asked him. *To be locked away in one of those places or to lose your life entirely?*

Robert thought about this. *It pains me to think of Jean falling victim to either of those fates.*

I would rather be dead than shut away, David said, decisively.

Angus look shocked and shook his head at his son. *It is not for you to choose. It is your duty to tell the truth and allow God to decide.*

David groaned. *It is not God who says what will happen to Jean. It is a group of men who look down on her because she is deaf and poor and a woman.*

Angus brought an outstretched right hand down onto his left palm. *If she tells the truth, God will protect her.*

David rolled his eyes. *How can you believe that? God cannot stop bad things befalling good people.*

Robert could see how frustrated David was becoming and he had a great deal of sympathy with the young man. He tried to explain the complexity of the situation. *I want to believe that God will look after her, but I have listened to what these men say about Jean. I think they want a resolution. I'm not sure they care about the truth. Forgive me, but if Jean insists on telling the truth, she may come to regret it.*

Angus regarded Robert. The minister seemed to be able to accept his son's rebellion against his doctrine, but he had not expected Robert to throw up his beliefs so readily.

'When you stand up in court, you will swear an oath on the Bible. Are you willing to betray that oath?' asked Angus. 'Because, believe you me, God will judge you for it. Would you lie and risk damnation for Jean Campbell?'

'I am there to interpret for her. I will do as I am bid.'

'And what if she says something you deem puts her in a dangerous situation? Will you be able to stop yourself relaying a sanitised version to the jury?'

David watched the two men talk until he grew so frustrated, he could bear it no longer. *Why have you both stopped signing? I have as much right as you both to know what is being said.*

I'm sorry. Robert apologised and did his best to relay in signs what he and Angus were arguing about.

Surely, you agree that Robert should defend her, David signed to his father.

Angus placed his teacup on its saucer and tried to explain. *Robert is not Jean's defence; he is her voice.* Angus pointed his index and middle finger towards his throat. *He must interpret her signs and gestures and render them into spoken English so that the court can hear both her plea and her testimony.*

This was a complicated concept for David to understand. The young man had never been inside a courtroom and had little notion of the way a trial was conducted.

So, he will tell them that the McDougalls are to blame for the death of her baby? David stated, as if there were no other logical course of action.

Robert sighed. *I cannot introduce evidence that doesn't exist.*

But Jean has told you what happened. You must tell the court.

Angus tried to defend why that couldn't happen. *Without any proof, Robert would simply be seen to be making wild allegations. If the court thinks that, he could be let go and then there would be no one to support Jean.*

David stared in disbelief at his father. *No! You've just said that he must interpret for Jean. So, if Jean tells the court what the McDougalls did to her child, Robert has to turn that into English for them.* David turned to Robert. *Is that not so?*

I suppose I must, Robert conceded. *But I can't help wondering if it would be better for Jean to say that the baby fell into the river by accident.*

Well, say that then. David sank back into his chair.

He can only say that if Jean signs it to him, Angus stated. He was as exasperated with his son as David was with what he saw as the ridiculousness of a situation in which the truth could not be heard.

Robert watched the young man and wondered at his own position. *Your father is right. I must speak to Jean and tell her of how things have gone here. We must both be clear about what we are going to tell the court and how.*

46

∼ Tuesday, 25 February 1817:
Partickhill Road, Glasgow ∼

Martha took a cloth and lifted one of the irons from the stove. She licked an index finger and tapped it on the iron's upturned base to make sure it was hot enough. She had already set two chairs back to back and now took a length of wood and balanced it between the chairs, smoothing a white baize ironing blanket over its surface.

A small, four-paned window in the scullery looked onto a path that ran along one side of the Partickhill villa. From her vantage point, Martha could see over some new hedging to a copse of trees beyond. She released the window catch, shoogled the upper part of the window and pulled it down as far as it would go. It had been raining and a faint smirr blew in and sprinkled her face. There were birds still calling from the trees even at this late hour.

Martha armed herself with the iron and began pressing one of the master's shirts. Yesterday, they had been steeped and washed and rinsed and hung outside, though the weather was still too cold to do the job properly. She didn't mind. Clothes were easier to iron when they were damp. She planned to air them on hangers overnight. Tomorrow, she would fold them neatly and take them upstairs to the master's bedroom, where she would place them carefully in a drawer, along with his bleached and starched collars.

A screech from outside pierced the silence. A fox, she thought.

Martha didn't mind being alone in the scullery in the late evenings. Ina had departed for the day and no one was likely to venture downstairs to disturb her. She was a maid inhabiting the servants' space and she felt safer here than anywhere else in the house. First thing in the morning and last thing at night she relished the chance to be alone, even though she continued to tend to the needs of others. Every portion of her time was packaged and tied like butcher's meat or lumps of cheese from the dairy.

It felt good to be released from the company of others. Ina was nice enough, but the old woman was her elder and better and knew more about every task involved in running a house; Martha constantly felt that her work would be judged and found wanting in some small way. Tonight, especially, she certainly didn't want to enter into any form of communication with either Mr McDougall or Dr Wilson. However, they were safely upstairs and were unlikely to come down. They might ring for her, but she could cope with that; there would be time to steady herself and, hopefully, it would only be because they wanted something to eat or drink or he'd need his bed turned down.

She swapped irons. The foxes were still at it. Fighting or mating. Those calls of theirs only happened in the darkness. Martha knew there were dens dotted about the hill, near the Hay Burn that ran south down to Partick. She had been told to chase the creatures if they came too close to the house, scavenging for scraps from the bins or the compost. She did so reluctantly. She liked the foxes. She sometimes caught sight of a vixen and her cubs. Once, she was cleaning out the privy and a cub bounded up to her. They regarded each other, both of them surprised at this unexpected meeting. Only when its mother stalked over, snarling, did the cub turn and run away. Ina had merely shrugged when she'd told her, uninterested in what had been, to Martha at least, a thrilling experience.

Martha had hoped that Ina wouldn't leave the house. She didn't fancy being alone here, with him. He had never bothered with her, seemed to see right through her, if anything, but she'd seen the way he treated his wife. Martha felt a twist in her stomach and struggled to push those images from her mind.

The clock in the front lobby struck eleven.

She perched the irons on the settle to cool and tidied up the scullery, closing the window again. In spite of the air coming in from outside, heat and steam fogged the room and rivulets of condensation ran down the plasterwork.

Martha blew out the candles, closed the doors to the kitchen and picked her way up the narrow back stairs. In the hallway, Dr Wilson's hat and coat were still on the coat stand, but she couldn't hear any voices coming from the drawing room, which seemed to be in darkness. She wondered if the master was up in his bedroom.

Martha continued to climb the stairs, trying to make as little noise as possible. Mrs McDougall was snoring in her bedroom, the doctor's bag still sitting just inside the doorway. Martha inched open the door that led up to the attic space in which she slept. The bare, wooden stairs that led the way were badly put together and creaked with every step.

~

Later, she lay quite still. If she worked in a bigger house, she might have had company. Another maid to swap stories and gossip with. Martha wondered what would happen to her next and prayed that Ina had been right, that her father had been told and that he would come to get her. She didn't want to stay here by herself.

If only she'd been sent to work in the pottery or at the weaving, but her parents thought this would be a better place. Service was more respectable; a job for life, or at least until she married – and you could sometimes live out once you had your own house and family. Her mother thought she'd be better off up the hill.

It had been alright for a while. She'd quite enjoyed going about the chores. The McDougalls had such nice things, it had been a pleasure to dust and polish them. Admire herself in her starched apron and cap; like a game of dressing-up.

After a few weeks though, the patina of respectability began to tarnish. Martha had always looked at these big houses and imagined that everyone inside would be warm and comfortable. But it soon became clear that the master and the mistress were far from happy, that all the blazing fires in the rooms and endless layers of soft woollen blankets could not keep them warm.

As more time passed, she heard raised voices and cleared away dishes from rooms where fury hung like a miasma around the silent and tense McDougalls. An unseen fist seemed to grip at Martha's chest and twist as she moved from below stairs to the public rooms on the ground floor of the villa and the private bedrooms and bathroom upstairs.

At bedtimes, she crept up the stairs as quietly as she could and slid the bolt on her bedroom door. She was glad she could lock it. She had heard terrible stories of girls in service whose bedrooms had no locks on them and of masters or other male servants who would creep in while they were sleeping and interfere with them. Her mother had always told her that if anyone tried to take liberties, she should scream and run home as fast as she could.

Now, she heard the master's low voice, steady and threatening. The scrape of a chair and the slam of a door.

Lots of men hit their wives. In that respect, the master wasn't unusual. It was the sober way he went about it that Martha found frightening; he never seemed overtaken by drink or an almighty passion like those men she had seen brawling with women in the streets or shouting from a house in the row of cottages where she had been brought up.

Mr McDougall was a gentleman. She had expected him to behave like one.

47

~ Friday, 14 March 1817:
The Tolbooth, Edinburgh ~

Robert slept late, surfacing only after midday. The previous day had been spent in travelling from Glasgow and, although he had tried to sleep inside the stage, his body had been jolted awake by every stone and divot on the highway. In addition, he could not shake the feeling of impotence that this latest trip to Glasgow had left him with.

He did not consider himself a proud man, but he had entertained hopes of returning to the capital with proof to back up Jean's story and, he was mortified to admit, imagined a scenario at the High Court where he might present his evidence and be hailed a hero of sorts. The reality of the situation was more mundane. It seemed that he now had little to offer either Jean or Lord Succoth; no villain of the piece and nothing concrete to show for what could now be considered merely a funded jaunt to the dear green place to peddle his wares. He felt like a fraud.

Still, the trial would go ahead, and he must now try to manage Jean's expectations and behaviour. It was important to minimise the damage to her and ensure that he was not complicit in ushering her to a fatal outcome. The best he could do now, he thought dejectedly, was to convince Jean to maintain that the baby's death had been accidental. If the worst then happened and she was found guilty, perhaps a manslaughter charge would save her from the noose.

~

Margaret had made up a posy from the garden for Jean and handed it to him as he left. *From my wife*, he signed as he handed the flowers to the prisoner in the Tolbooth's cell, making a handshape to represent the placing of a wedding ring on someone's finger.

Jean smiled as she took them from him and placed them in a tumbler by the narrow window where a crack of light was permitted entry to the room. They both stood for a few moments looking at the sprigs of flowers and leaves; cheerful yellow stars of celandine, white petals that burst on sprays of ivy and the soft compact furs of pussy willow. Tiny harbingers of a spring that was revealing itself to the world outside. Robert wondered if the blossom would last until the end of the trial. He glanced at Jean and wondered if she were thinking the same thing.

Your wife keeps well?

Very well, thank you.

She is not sick? Jean made a vomiting gesture with both her hands and Robert looked at her, confused as to what she meant.

With the baby?

He laughed and shook his head. *She was sick before, but not now. A little tired, still.*

Jean nodded and smiled. *This is what happens. I am glad she is well and that your child grows inside her.*

Robert coloured. He felt embarrassed. The conflation of his two worlds made him uncomfortable. The fact that Margaret had bade him take the flowers and Jean's interest in this, still private, aspect of his domestic life. And yet, at the same time, it made the prospect of his becoming a father real and that pleased him.

Sit down. Please. He motioned to her.

You have been to Glasgow? Jean asked.

He nodded. *I have. I tried my best to find someone to bear*

241

witness to your story, but I am sorry to tell you I have failed. The McDougalls are no longer in their house and I cannot find out where either of them have gone.

The minister and his family, they could not help you?

Quite the opposite. They did all they could. Robert indicated the Buchanans' efforts by motioning his palms at right angles to each other. *David even came with me to Partickhill to look for McDougall but no one there knows where he has gone.*

It is like chasing ghosts. Jean held her hands together and then pulled them apart, indicating a vanishing act.

Yes, he agreed, *every time I got close to finding them, they seemed to disappear. I did meet the young woman who you knew in the house. The maid. I found her at her parents' house down by the river in Partick.*

Jean brightened. *She no longer works for them?*

No. She has found work elsewhere. She said to tell you she sends her good wishes. She wanted me to give you this.

Robert reached into the pocket of his greatcoat and brought out the white cotton cap that Martha had given him. Jean's breath caught in her throat as she recognised it. She took it from him and laid it on her lap. She began to cry in gulps of pain, the magnitude of her loss concentrated in this scant fragment of material.

I'm so sorry, Robert said, reaching out a hand to take the cap back again. *I didn't mean to upset you.*

Jean shook her head and held the little cap tightly. *I'm glad of it. It was kind of her to think enough of me to keep it safe.*

Martha was distressed about what had happened to you. She wanted to help but knew nothing of the whereabouts of the McDougalls. She did not see what happened in that room and she seemed frightened, perhaps was too frightened to say anything against them even if she was able to.

Jean's mouth twitched, as if she were attempting a smile

but had not the heart for it. *I am glad she's safe. I would not wish that man's violence on anyone.*

Even on his wife? Robert asked.

I would wish my own violence on that bitch.

What do you mean? What has his wife done to you?

Jean stared at him but said nothing. Robert averted his eyes but steeled himself to continue.

Which of them killed your child? Was it McDougall, or was it his wife?

He just cleaned up afterwards. Tried to kill me. You know who it was.

If you tell me, we can find a way to get you out of here.

Jean sighed. *You said yourself, they are nowhere to be found. He has spirited her away, hidden her so that she can't answer for what she has done, and he can pretend to be the injured party.*

Robert threw up his hands. *No. Don't you see? What matters is making sure the jury can't find you guilty. Charles and Euphemia McDougall are not my concern now. Perhaps they will get their just deserts in this life, perhaps not. God will judge them, though, and he will find them wanting. Their punishment will be meted out beyond the grave.*

Do you believe that? Jean asked him.

I do, Robert said. *We are all of us answerable for our actions. If, for whatever reason, our fellow men do not hold us to account then God will surely do it on judgement day.*

48

∼ Saturday, 15 March 1817:
Chessels Court, Edinburgh ∼

Margaret stirred her tea and looked at Robert thoughtfully.

'In the meantime, you still need to make sure she gets away with it,' she said. 'God might want you to atone on judgement day, Robbie, did you ever consider that?'

'I'm not helping her to get away with anything, I'm trying to control what she tells the court. The simpler her story the better.'

'You mean, if the court think she's simple-minded because she's deaf, they might just believe that she didn't mean to cause the death of her baby.'

Robert sighed, but he nodded.

'It's not exactly the favourable perception of deaf people that you've been trying to promote all this time, is it?' she said, more as an observation than a criticism.

'No, it's not,' he agreed.

Robert lifted his cup to his lips but did not drink. Instead, he placed it back on its saucer and studied the knots and grooves in the surface of the long kitchen table.

'I wish I'd never been called in on this case, Maggie. I am in an impossible position. I cannot tell the truth because no one will believe Jean's story without evidence. If I allow her to tell it regardless, it will be treated as the ranting of a madwoman and she might be locked away for good. The best we can hope for now is that she gives the jury the bare minimum and they think it was an accident.'

'You've done your best, Robbie. You should not expect any more of yourself.'

'I wanted to prove her innocence, and I wanted to prove that the deaf are the same as the hearing. That their stories deserve to be heard.'

'I know.'

'I thought I could achieve something on their behalf,' said Robert.

Margaret poured them both another cup of tea. 'You still can. You can achieve something on Jean's behalf. You have some power over this situation. The person who interprets Jean's plea and testimony is in control of what is communicated to the court.'

'But I am sworn to tell the truth, the whole truth and nothing but the truth.'

Margaret shook her head. 'Don't you see? Jean is sworn to do that. You, on the other hand, are sworn to report what she signs to you.'

'You talk of control as if I can choose what parts of her testimony I relay. If I am sworn to give an accurate interpretation, I must do that. It would still be a sin to alter anything.'

'We both know that interpreting signs is not an exact science. There are nuances, there are ambiguities that do not shift from signing to speech in the same way and to the same extent that they do from one written language to another.'

'How is that relevant, though?'

'You are an interpreter, Robbie. You're not a translator. What you do is take apart a deaf person's signs and allow them to reassemble as speech. You don't present a facsimile. That would be impossible. It's like a piece of knitting or dress-making that doesn't quite fit the person it's intended for; you unravel it and rework it until it does.

And what's more, nobody in that courtroom, perhaps excepting myself, will be able to see where you deviate from the pattern.'

'I have to interpret in good faith. I cannot deviate on purpose.'

Margaret rolled her eyes. 'You worry too much. God will understand.'

Robert gave a rueful laugh. 'God will judge me if I lie.'

'I'll absolve you, Robbie. Let me be your conscience.'

'That's a blasphemous thing to say.'

She laughed. 'It's a practical thing to say.'

49

∽ Monday, 17 March 1817:
The High Court, Edinburgh ∽

Laymen and members of the public attending trials at the Scottish Court of High Justiciary were required to enter the building through the main doorway at Parliament Square. Once inside, the large lobby thronged with people. Some, dressed in the black gowns of the legal profession, were intent and purposeful, familiar with the machinations of the building and its inhabitants. Others, who were there as witnesses to the numerous cases on trial at any one time, stood around hesitantly, trying to identify a source of information that might point them in the right direction.

The courtroom in which Jean's trial was to be heard was on the first floor. On his arrival at the court, Robert had located Succoth's senior writer, Archibald Gibson, who had, in turn, given him into the care of a young clerk. Robert followed the boy up a stone staircase, past paintings of robed men rendered gloomily in oils. Inside the court-room itself, each wall was panelled in ponderous oak to the halfway point. Above this the walls were covered in horse-hair plaster and, on one side, there were rows of windows that were so elevated that all that could be seen through them were bleached oblongs of sky.

Groups of men bustled around carrying sheaves of papers, their cloaks flapping and shoes click-clacking, mustering like a murder of crows. They were enacting a peculiar theatre, unintelligible to outsiders.

The various people who were crowded into the room for the trial had been sitting there for some considerable time, waiting patiently while the administrative business of the court was organised.

Robert shuffled on the narrow bench where he had been instructed to wait until his name was called. He craned his neck to see what was happening in the main body of the court. He wanted to find out if Margaret had arrived but, tucked behind a partition, he could only see the front of the court where Lord Succoth sat, surveying tables full of lawyers and clerks.

The spectators were there, though; audible both above and behind him. Robert fiddled with his good cravat, which was both too tight and too starchy. Being dressed in his best clothes should have lent him some confidence but, paradoxically, only served to make him more nervous.

Eventually, Succoth called the court to order. He explained that the trial of Jean Campbell would go ahead if it could be established to the court's satisfaction that she was a fit person to be examined.

Robert was ushered from the bench and brought round into the courtroom proper, where he sat behind the table with the defence lawyer and his assistants. A door opened to the side of the room and Jean was led in. She disappeared behind Robert and he wondered if she were now sat on the narrow bench, waiting to be summoned.

Edwin Browne was the first of the three experts to be called. He took the stand and reiterated what Robert recalled him saying previously and privately; that, apart from a defect in hearing, Jean was a satisfactorily healthy specimen of her sex and class.

Succoth thanked him and instructed the clerk to call the next witness.

'Gentlemen of the jury,' Succoth began, 'you are now

to hear the expert testimony of Dr Jeremiah Pringle. Dr Pringle is Professor in Moral Philosophy at the University of Edinburgh. He has no direct knowledge of the events that took place on February twenty-fourth in Glasgow, save that the prisoner is charged with the murder of a child on that date. Dr Pringle is asked to give his opinion as to the efficacy of examining a deaf and dumb prisoner. In particular, whether, as such an individual, Jean Campbell is intellectually suited to stand trial. There is an additional consideration in respect of this question – even if the accused is able to give coherent answers, can she be made sufficiently aware of the deliberations of this court-room to appreciate what is happening?'

Jeremiah Pringle, who had been standing next to the clerk in the doorway, approached the witness box and took the stand.

'Dr Pringle,' Succoth said, 'can you tell the court what your contact has been with the prisoner thus far?'

Pringle pursed his lips, blinked, and began, 'It was requested that I meet with the prisoner and consult with Your Lordship on the advisability of prosecuting the prisoner on the charge of murder.'

'And that was immediately after the panel was arrested, is that correct?' Succoth asked.

'Yes, Your Lordship. The prisoner had been brought to Edinburgh from Glasgow, where the authorities were at a loss as to how to deal with her.'

'Why was that, Dr Pringle?'

'Well, they had a crime and a prisoner, but no way of examining her. She is deaf and dumb and did not answer to those who spoke to her. There was an assumption, an entirely understandable one, that she was incapable of communicating. It seemed that she would have to be dealt with as an imbecile or an idiot.'

Succoth nodded. 'Can you explain to the court what that means?'

Pringle nodded in turn. 'This category of people, should they be guilty of a crime, are not tried in open court but given over to the stewardship of the local asylum.'

'If I recall correctly,' said Succoth, 'was there not some doubt on the part of the Glasgow police as to what was the most advisable course of action in the case of Jean Campbell?'

'Yes, it would appear so. They requested a transfer to Edinburgh in order that her condition be assessed.'

'They were not convinced that Jean Campbell was suffering from insanity or idiocy?'

Pringle shook his head. 'They found themselves unable to determine that, Your Lordship.'

'And what did you find when you interviewed the panel?'

'At our initial meeting, very little. I established that she is deaf and dumb and communicates primarily by the use of signs. I could not understand her and was unable, there-fore, to make any definitive judgement as to her fitness to plead. However, my first impressions were of a woman of no little self-possession. I felt it would be appropriate to consult someone with a knowledge of her language in order that she might be questioned further.'

'How did you go about that?' Succoth asked.

'I recommended that we call in the teacher at the Deaf and Dumb Institution in the Canongate, Mr Robert Kinniburgh. Once Kinniburgh had interviewed the panel, an informed judgement could be made as to her ability to plead.'

'Can you tell this court what your subsequent conclusions were?'

'The panel was distressed about the fate of her baby.

She professed some horror that the child was dead. When Mr Kinniburgh told her that she was accused of wilful murder of her own child, she became entirely distraught. She denied it in the strongest of terms, repeatedly and forcefully.'

Succoth nodded. 'Are you satisfied, Dr Pringle, that Jean Campbell understands that she is on trial for murder?'

'I am,' Pringle confirmed.

'Do you believe that Jean Campbell is of sufficient intelligence to understand the difference between right and wrong?'

'Yes. In fact, I believe that the panel's feelings of moral abhorrence may well be more vivid than those of the ordinary person, who is able to hear the language of ruffianism. She has no education to speak of, but she is vociferous in declaiming her innocence. I cannot help but be convinced of her ability to distinguish between a moral and an immoral act.'

Succoth thanked Dr Pringle and then explained that, as Jean was deaf and dumb, any testimony made by her would have to be translated into the language that the court could understand, much in the same way as anyone with a foreign tongue would be handled by the justiciary.

A clerk called out Jean's name and she was led to the witness box. She was soberly dressed in Maggie's linen gown and dark bonnet.

Succoth asked Robert to approach the bench.

'Mr Kinniburgh, you are the teacher at the Deaf and Dumb Institution in Edinburgh, is that correct?'

'Yes, my Lord.'

'And would you consider yourself to be proficient in the language of the deaf and dumb?

'I would, Your Lordship.'

'Very well. Do you swear to give a just and true

interpretation of the prisoner's account of the events of the twenty-fourth of February this year?'

'I do.'

Succoth motioned to Robert to approach the prisoner. 'You must explain the oath to her, Mr Kinniburgh.'

Robert looked at Jean. He pointed above his head and then sliced his right hand down onto the flat of his left palm.

Do you swear to tell the truth, in front of God?

Jean nodded.

'The accused swears the oath, my Lord.'

Robert and Jean shared a glance. The courtroom was silent, the anticipation of the spectators bearing down on them. I am the only one who knows your story, thought Robert, I must relay it to the best of my abilities. I have sworn before God to give a just and true interpretation of your account. I have not sworn to tell the truth.

Robert began by asking Jean to state her name and her place of birth and relayed that to the bench.

Lord Succoth instructed him to explain to Jean what the court needed to know from her.

I must now ask you about the crime you are accused of. Do you understand?

Jean nodded.

He then made a figure with his handkerchief across his left arm in imitation of the baby lying there. Standing at the bar, he made a sign with his right hand, as if he were throwing the figure or baby over it, purposely away from himself. He made a sign resembling the winding water of the river and then, suddenly, a more violent sign. Robert flattened the palm of his right hand and brought it sharply to his forehead.

Did you throw the child into the river? Did you kill your baby?

Jean stared coolly at him; her face betrayed no emotion. *No. I did not.*

Robert turned to Succoth.

'The panel pleads Not Guilty, my Lord.'

~

There was a flurry of people and papers. Some left the courtroom, and yet more entered it. Succoth introduced the counsel for the prosecution. 'If you're ready, Mr McCormack?'

McCormack, a tall reed of a man who seemed to still be outgrowing his clothes, called his first witness. This was a skinny, snottery lad named George Monteith, who looked to be between fourteen and fifteen years of age. Being sworn, McCormack began his questioning.

'Mr Monteith, can you give the court your recollection of the events of the twenty-fourth of February?'

Monteith said that he remembered seeing the prisoner on the Old Bridge but was not absolutely sure of the time, although it was dark, so must have been in the late afternoon or early evening. He was on his way to his brother's house at the Bridge-end and spotted the prisoner near Clark's eating house at the Briggait. She had a bundle tied to her breast by means of a scarf or a shawl. He assumed it was a small child but hadn't actually had sight of it.

McCormack looked confused and scrutinised the witness from over the top of his pince-nez.

'You didn't know what was in the bundle the panel was carrying?'

'No, sir, not then, but a few seconds later I noticed the same woman on the opposite side of the bridge to me.'

'What was she doing?' asked McCormack.

'I wasn't entirely sure,' the boy answered. 'She had her

253

back to me and was leaning on the parapet of the bridge. She stumbled and held on to it for support. I thought she might be a beggar woman. I was worried she might be fu' so I took care to avoid her in case she tried to tap me.'

McCormack affected an expression of deep consideration, as if he were solving a complicated riddle. 'You thought she was intoxicated and worried she might accost you for money?'

'Aye,' replied Monteith.

McCormack nodded his satisfaction and gestured to the lad to carry on.

'When I reached the north side of the river, I turned left in the direction of my brother's house and I heard a shout and saw a baby falling into the water.'

'How far away from the panel were you?' asked McCormack.

Monteith thought for a moment.

'Perhaps only a fathom's length, sir?'

'You're quite sure it was a child?'

Monteith nodded. 'I feel sure it was. I saw the dress and the figure of it.'

'Was it alive? Did its body move, or perhaps it was the child that you heard cry out?'

'It didn't sound like the cry of a child, sir. I couldn't say for certain if it was alive or dead as it fell. It disappeared so quickly into the water.'

'Did you hear a splash as it hit the water?'

'I don't recall hearing much of a noise at all.'

'What happened after the bundle, whether it was indeed a baby or not, fell into the water?'

'I saw an old man approach the panel on the bridge. He seemed to be comforting her. Then two bakers came up to me and I told them that I had seen the woman throw a child over the bridge. One of the bakers went to fetch the police and the other ran down to the edge of the water to see if the child was still visible. I followed this second man; in case we might spot the poor child and be able to rescue it.'

McCormack paused, then looked towards the jury as he posed his next question.

'Was there any sign of the poor little creature?'

George Monteith shook his head.

Lord Succoth interjected, 'Speak up, lad.'

'We couldn't see anything, Your Lordship. I followed the baker down the embankment, but it was pitch dark down there. We tore a branch from a tree, and I held one end while the baker held the other and waded some way into the water.'

'Did you see what happened to the woman on the bridge?' McCormack asked.

'When we scrambled up to the top of the embankment again, I saw the police sergeant running towards the toll-house at the foot of the Briggait. The old man and some other people had seized the lady who is now your prisoner and were also walking towards the tollhouse.'

'Did you speak to the police sergeant?' McCormack asked.

George Monteith shook his head. 'Not then, sir. By the time we had righted ourselves and made to follow in that direction, the police sergeant was escorting the woman towards the jail. I couldn't get into the police office on account of the crowd that had gathered. The next day, I was examined in the City Chambers and gave a report of what I'd seen.'

McCormack dismissed George Monteith and called Archibald Angus, another passer-by who had seen Jean Campbell at the Old Bridge.

Robert glanced over in Jean's direction. She looked preternaturally calm. Her bearing seemed at odds with the witness's account of events. Robert wondered what the jury thought of her. Would they judge her on perceived reactions even though they must know she couldn't hear what was being discussed? He caught her eye and inclined his head slightly, trying to convey something, he knew not what. He wished he were able to interpret the witness statements for her but that had not been deemed necessary. He would try to remember the gist of what was said and relay it to her later in the Tolbooth. Robert looked around the courtroom and saw Margaret sitting amongst the spectators, her head inclined to one side as she watched Monteith leave and the next witness appear by the same door.

Archibald Angus was a stocky young man of about twenty. He had been crossing over from north to south in the direction of Laurieston at about a quarter past five that fateful evening. He remembered seeing the prisoner reclining on the bridge and looking into the water.

'Was she holding anything, Mr Angus?'

'Not as far as I could see, sir.'

'Did you notice her throw anything from the bridge?'

'No, but she had her back to me.'

'I see,' said McCormack. 'What is your recollection of what happened next?'

'I saw a lad, who I know now to be the witness George Monteith, run towards two men who were approaching the bridge. The lights from the shops on the north side of the river illuminated them for a moment and then they disappeared from sight. I turned back to see where the woman had gone as she seemed in some distress. I saw the police sergeant appear followed by a group of people, who seized her, near the tollhouse, and took her to the police office.'

McCormack nodded.

'Thank you, Mr Angus.'

Lord Succoth then called John McLeod, the police sergeant who had been on duty that evening and who Robert had met in Glasgow.

'Sergeant McLeod,' McCormack began, 'can you tell the court what happened after you seized the prisoner on the night in question?'

'I took her round to the police office, sir, and I tried to take down her name and other particulars, as is usually the case when someone is arrested,' McLeod replied in his faint Highland accent.

'But that wasn't possible with Jean Campbell?'

The police sergeant shook his head. 'No. After a short time, I was told that she was deaf and dumb and, although I wrote down the questions that I needed her to answer, it was obvious that she couldn't read either. Eventually, I just put her in a cell and waited until later when I got some help from a deaf fellow that worked locally.'

'And what help did this man give you?'

'None, if truth be told, sir. He was willing enough and he did his best by making signs, but Jean Campbell couldn't, or wouldn't, talk to him. We were stuck, sir, if you see what I'm saying.'

'I believe she has another child,' McCormack stated. 'A son. He was brought to the police office shortly after her arrest?'

'Yes, sir. A lad of about six years, sir,' McLeod answered.

'And was the son able to speak to his mother? Was he deaf and dumb as well?'

'No, sir. He could hear perfectly well. I let him see his mother in the hope that she might tell him something, but the wee boy just became confused and upset. His mother looked quite wretched. I didn't feel there was anything to be gained by keeping him there.'

'What happened to him?'

'I believe a gentleman from the parish came to collect the boy.'

McCormack affected a look of bemusement. 'And you simply let him go?'

'I was occupied with the prisoner. When she calmed down and I got her into a cell, the boy had already gone.'

'Had he been taken to the poorhouse?'

'That's what I assumed, sir.'

'Do you know where the boy is now?'

'No, sir, I don't.'

'And we have no testimony from him?'

'We do not, sir.'

McCormack sighed and made a pantomime of disappointment, but McLeod was used to the play-acting of lawyers and kept his countenance steady, and his mouth firmly shut.

Lord Succoth raised his hand.

'Mr McCormack, this boy is aged around five or six years old. I can't imagine that his recall of an event that happened close to a month ago will be of any use to us now. It's debatable whether it would have been of use on the night itself.'

'Excuse me, my Lord,' said McCormack, 'I was just curious as to why he had not been questioned by the officer.'

Succoth sighed. 'I doubt he'd have had anything to add.'

The final witness for the prosecution was Mr Duncan, the boatman from the Glasgow Humane Society, who had spent so long searching for the child's body. Mr Duncan was a stout man who wore a weather-beaten aspect. He entered the courtroom and bustled forwards to take the stand. As he gave his testimony, he twisted a plaid bunnet in his hands and told the court about the difficulties he had encountered. He explained the vagaries of tides and weather and expressed his deep sense of regret that he had not been successful.

The court broke for the day and Robert went outside. The rain was still beating down, coursing along a higgledy-piggledy network of drainpipes and splashing into the gutters between pavement and street. There he found Maggie, sheltering under the overhang of a statue. They picked their way along to the nearest coffee house, where they ordered two bowls of thin vegetable soup and looked out desultorily at the sodden city.

50

~ Monday, 24 February 1817:
The Old Bridge, Glasgow ~

Jean's flight from the house in Partickhill was a journey of three distinct stages. Down to Partick, then along the river into the city, and finally, an attempt to reach Taylor's Close. Even in the chaos of leaving, her instinct was to return to a place she knew and where there would be people who could help her.

She held the baby's lifeless body to her as she approached the Dumbarton Road. The closer she got to the thorough-fare, the more people there were. Some walking along intent on a destination, others juking across in front of carts and carriages to get to the opposite side or stopping to talk to acquaintances or enter a close or shop.

His body was wrapped in the shawl she had been wearing about her shoulders. She folded herself around this shape and determined not to let it go.

He had not been baptised in any church. Jean understood that he ought to have been given a legitimate name. Her ownership of him could be disputed and he might not be given a proper burial. She had to get him to safety, find the minister and ask what must be done to save her poor son's soul.

She headed south in the direction of the river. Shops and taverns gave way to streets where there was mainly industry. Coils of rope piled high and barrels outside a cooperage. Red sparks flying from a blacksmith's forge as horses stamped and railed against the confined quarters in which they found themselves.

An image of Mrs McDougall's face, full of spiteful glee, swam in front of Jean and made her dizzy. She pushed it away and stopped to steady herself, taking great gulps of air to propel herself forward.

Eventually she turned a corner and saw an expanse of water in front of her, small ships and boats jostling for position between Partick and the quays on the Govan side of the Clyde. There was a sharp east wind blowing and the clouds were darkening. She shivered without her shawl.

~

Mr McDougall emerged from his wife's bedroom and flew out of the house in only his shirtsleeves. No hat or coat. From the kitchen, Ina heard him slam the front door. Martha was shaking silently, too shocked to cry.

Martha had tried to stop Jean from leaving with the wee one but the deaf woman, exhausted as she was, seemed to have the strength of a prize fighter and pushed her roughly out the way. Martha had fallen backwards and lost her balance, landing awkwardly on her hip, which hurt like blazes. Still, she didn't blame Jean. The poor woman had been frantic.

Martha was finding it hard to make sense of everything; the expression on Mrs McDougall's face as she snatched the baby from Jean and his cries that so abruptly stopped. Had there been some kind of accident? Surely, no one could have meant to kill the wee boy? She simply didn't know what to think anymore. Then there was the master; he had looked ready to do violence when he realised that Jean had left the house with the baby's body. There was something in this house, she thought, something evil and twisted. It had infected everyone in it.

Ina appeared by her side. 'Is he away?' she asked.

'Yes,' said Martha. 'Do you think he's gone to find Jean?'

'I don't know, hen. I hope not.' Ina put her arm around Martha's shoulders. 'We cannae do anything for Jean now, hen. We'd better go upstairs and see to the mistress.'

'What do you think he's done to her?' the girl asked, fearfully.

Ina shrugged and began to climb the stairs. In spite of her trepidation, Martha followed her.

~

Mrs McDougall was crouched, hunched up in the window recess in her bedroom. A mass of bruising flowering on one side of her face. A patch of hair matted and damp with blood. Her blank eyes resting on nothing.

Martha's gaze dropped and she took in the mistress's fingers, next to a pool of sticky blood, some of which had been smeared on the wall and skirting board.

'Jesus,' Ina said, softly.

Ina looked like she was about to weep but, instead, sat down on the top of the tangle of sheets and blankets that half covered the bed. Martha stood by helplessly. She awaited the older woman's instructions, unsure if they would ever come. Ina, usually so capable, looked completely spent. Martha wished beyond anything that she could go home and be with her mother and father in the noisy, cramped cottage at Castlebank Street.

Eventually, Ina drew herself up and went over to Mrs McDougall. The mistress flinched when the cook touched her arm.

'It's alright, hen,' Ina whispered. 'You're safe with me. Let me help you get into your bed. You'll be comfier there.'

Ina indicated to Martha to square up the bedclothes and slowly Mrs McDougall was brought to her feet. Her dress was marked and torn, and Martha walked over to the recess to pick up one of the mistress's slippers that had fallen there. As she bent down, she spotted two broken pieces of tooth wedged into the crack between floorboards and her breath caught in her throat. She picked them up carefully and deposited the teeth into the pocket of her pinny.

The mistress's face was bad but there was also bruising at her arms where McDougall had dug his fingers in as he gripped her.

'Bastard's an animal,' muttered Ina as she manoeuvred Mrs McDougall onto the bed. She began to unbutton what was left of the mistress's clothes, taking them off as gently as she was able, then handing the articles to Martha. When Mrs McDougall was down to her underclothes, Ina checked her over and, wringing out a cloth on the washstand, cleaned up the blood as best she could.

'Should I go and fetch the doctor?' Martha asked.

'Not yet,' said Ina. 'I'll give her a sleeping draught. Go and get a tumbler of brandy out of the good decanter in the dining room for to wash it down. We might as well let her get some rest. God knows when the master will be back.'

~

By the time Charles reached the outskirts of the city, evening was creeping in. Despite having come out in such an almighty hurry, he still had his pocketbook with him and could have hailed a carriage to take him all the way to the Saltmarket. But, not wanting to draw attention to himself, he had kept his head down and trudged along the riverside on foot.

It had been years since he had walked all the way into the city. As a young man he had undertaken this length of journey often, sometimes tramping from dawn to call at hiring places the length of the Clyde, getting a full day's work and walking, tired and hungry, back to his lodgings at Kelvinhaugh. He had always kept to the north side of the river, not wanting to venture south to the Gorbals or Tradeston. Knowing no one there, he preferred to stick to his stamping grounds of Partick or the Broomielaw, places where he was a fairly well kent face and might have a chance to jump the queue for any available work.

Today, he wished that he could again clothe himself in the anonymity he had so gratefully shrugged off as he climbed the ladder from casual labourer to successful shipyard owner.

Charles stopped at an inn on Cheapside Street and ordered a hauf and a hauf. A mirror above the bar, silvered by time, showed his reflection. He saw a man who looked as if he had been brawling in the street or been tumbled for money. His hair stood up wildly and there were scratches on his cheek where Euphemia had tried to claw at him. He took his drink and sat down at an empty space in a corner, hoping it would afford him some cover, and tried not to draw attention to himself. As he picked up the drinks, he noticed that his hands were shaking and, much as he craved the solace of alcohol, he found it hard to swallow the liquid down.

He had to find that deaf hoor and get the baby's body from her. If she went to the police with a story of murder and mayhem, it was possible she would be believed. At the very least, the police might take an interest in him and his household. That was the last thing Charles wanted. Who knows what the old cook and the girl might say if questioned? And God forbid Euphemia should be given a voice. A man had dominion over his wife, but Charles did not trust his own to keep some aspects of their relationship private.

Charles knew Jean had lived with the taig, Donnelly, near Merchants' Hall and his intention was to track her as far as the Green. If he hadn't found her by then, he would have to return home and reconsider his position. The doctor would need to be consulted on what to do with Euphemia. He could try to pay off the servants and keep them quiet that way, but Euphemia was not so easily bought. Keeping her medicated on a constant basis wasn't practically – or financially – viable.

He sipped at his whisky. All of these possibilities were nothing compared to finding that woman and the baby and making sure no one else found them first.

He must press on.

~

Jean crouched in a doorway off the Broomielaw. The rain had come on heavy and she needed to shelter from it. She also needed to rest. The burst of energy that had spurred her on was beginning to fail her now. The wind swept sheets of rain into the doorway and moisture settled on her woollen skirt. She tucked her legs underneath her. It was quiet here. One or two pedestrians had walked past but they hadn't paid her any attention. In their hurry to escape the weather, a poor woman hunched up against the elements was not worth remarking upon. If they had the time to linger, they might only have noticed that she was holding a sleeping baby.

The rags between her legs felt heavy. She had been bleeding, on and off, since the birth, and now she visualised them sodden with blood and her stomach heaved. She hadn't eaten for hours and, even then, it had only been a slice of toast and jam at breakfast. They had finished that repast quickly, she and Martha, having other things to do.

She didn't recognise him at first. Her attention was caught purely by the rapidity of his walking and the fact that his clothes were simultaneously expensive and dishevelled. The usual type of man who walked by wore boots, waistcoat, frock coat and a bowler or a broad cap. The colour in their clothes bleached by constant wear. Respectable but drab. Charles McDougall, in contrast, was dressed in shirtsleeves and formal checked trousers but had no head covering or necktie. As he came closer, she realised who he was and flinched.

Jean gathered her skirt around her and shrank into the corner of the doorway. It stank of piss, but she buried her head in the shawl that wrapped the baby's body and breathed in his smell, fervently hoping that McDougall wouldn't notice her.

She kept watch from the corner of her eye until he crossed the road and disappeared out of sight. Peeking out from her hiding place, she followed his journey as he carried on along the riverside. He could only be pursuing her. Why else would he be in this neighbourhood dressed so strangely? He was heading in the same direction that she had been, so she decided to change tack.

Jean's heart was racing again. She pulled herself upright and clutched the bundle to her. She stumbled as she stepped onto the pavement and had to steady herself against the wall of the building. But soon she was on the move again, propelled forward by a force she seemed to have no control over. She would cross the river and come at the Saltmarket by the opposite direction. It would take longer, but it would mean she could keep an eye out for McDougall, and hopefully he would have been and gone by the time she arrived in Taylor's Close. He knew no one there and a man of his social standing would be given short shrift by the locals if he began asking questions about her.

~

When she had crossed the river by the wooden bridge, she hesitated, not wanting to walk along the pristine pavement at Carlton Place. She clambered down the embankment and began to follow a rough path that meandered along between the riverbed and a high stone wall that shored up the land where the new houses had been built.

Jean felt simultaneously numb and sore. Her mind was empty, focused only on getting to Taylor's Close. But the aches and pains were all too prevalent; the flight into the city had completely disturbed a body that ought to have been resting.

All at once, she was caught by an arm across her chest and another grabbing her by the waist. The baby's body in his tightly wrapped bundle fell towards the ground, the shawl unwrapping as she was wrenched away from him. She could smell McDougall's sweat and cologne, mingling together.

Charles's arm around her was so tight that she couldn't move, and he edged her downwards and on the wet grass. Her hand was trapped but her fingers stretched out in the direction that the baby had fallen.

He forced her down, until she was lying on the ground,

her cheek pressed against the muddy grass, howling into the earth as he leant all his weight upon her to keep her quiet. Charles's breath was hot and sharp at her neck and she could feel his lips move as if he were saying something to her, but she couldn't tell what.

He pushed against her in a strange simulation of the sexual act and, in her confused state, she wondered if that was what he was about to do. She knew of men who took great pride in having slept with women who had not long given birth; who staked their claim over them so that they knew not to prize their children over their husbands. Jealous, violent men just like the kind she had discovered Charles McDougall to be. She started to cry, tears covering her face, mingling with rain-drenched leaves.

Then, abruptly, he turned her round and pulled himself up awkwardly to a sitting position astride her, using his knees to pin her arms at her sides as he did so. His face was red and sore, scratches at his eyes. She wondered who had done that. Had it been his bitch of a wife or had she done it herself? She couldn't remember. She wasn't sure what was happening anymore or if she were awake or dreaming. She was in pain. She was light-headed. Charles's hands were pushing down on her windpipe. Spit dribbled from his mouth onto her face, all his energy concentrated in his task. She could feel herself drifting in and out of consciousness and she knew he was trying to kill her, but she could do nothing about it. Her eyes closed and she went limp.

Charles loosened his grip, panting, Jean's body beneath him. He slowly became aware of his surroundings again and the fear of being discovered returned. As he began to push himself up, he wasn't aware of Jean's knee moving. She jerked it upwards and caught him square in the groin. With her free arms she grabbed his face and thrust her thumbs into his eyes. He rolled down the embankment, howling in pain.

This was all Jean needed to rally again. She stood up and kicked him as hard as she could as they both fumbled for her dead child's body. She got to the baby first and, as Charles tried to stand up, the pain in his groin caught him unawares and he slipped back down the muddy embankment towards the riverbed.

Jean was disorientated. It was dark now, but she wasn't sure if it was cloudy or evening or if her eyesight had simply become blurred as a result of the assault she had just been subjected to.

She ran up towards the roadside in the direction of the Old Bridge. There was nobody around so she kept moving, trying to put as much distance between herself and Charles as she could. But an overwhelming need to vomit overtook her and she bent over, her stomach emptying itself of what little she had eaten that day. Her throat felt like it was full of broken glass, so narrow she could hardly take a breath.

Again, she felt Charles's hand was on her shoulder, but there was a lack of purchase, he was weaker than before. She jammed her elbow into his ribs and started running. But this spurt of energy took her no further than the middle of the Old Bridge before she was forced to stop and try to catch her breath again. Her windpipe felt as if it were collapsing in on itself. Her vision was blurred and intermittent. She pushed a hand forward to steady herself on the wooden parapet of the bridge. But she misjudged the distance and tumbled forward, and the bundle of material that contained her baby's body first lurched from her hold and then fell over the edge of the bridge, plummeting down into the dirty water below.

She cried out, weakly, hoarsely, but it echoed in the still evening and the sound travelled. To the south, where

Charles was standing at the Gorbals side, and to the north, where a trickle of people made their way along the Briggait.

Charles McDougall at first made to reach her but, on hearing a cry go up from the opposite bank, collected himself and retreated into the darkness.

51

Charles sat at his desk; shoulders hunched. He merged into the surroundings of the darkened room.

There was no fire lighted, no candles burning. The people of the house had other work to do.

From the room above, floorboards creaked. Charles heard the bell ring and Martha's footsteps hurry up the stairs. He poked at the inside of his nostrils with a finger, picking away the grime that had collected there. He searched in his pocket for a handkerchief, then wiped his finger on his trousers in the absence of one. He gagged as he remembered that he had used it in an attempt to mop up the infant's blood.

There had been a lot of blood and the handkerchief had not been sufficient to the task. Charles remembered throwing the soaked cotton square into the fire in an impotent rage, watching it sit limply there, the saturated blood refusing to catch fire. Everything, even the most basic of elements, against him.

There was a tentative knock at the door.

Dr Wilson looked guarded as he stepped inside the room. The lamps were burning in the rest of the house and it took his eyes a few moments to adjust to the gloom. He walked over to a pair of winged armchairs arranged in the bay of the window and slumped down on one. He leant his elbows on the armrests and rubbed at his temples.

'I've made her comfortable,' he said. The doctor's voice was a monotone, his expression blank.

'It's more than the bitch deserves,' Charles snarled. 'She's lucky she's not locked up in a cell at the police office.'

The lack of light in the room hid the splashes of mud on Charles's clothes and the dishevelled aspect that his pursuit of Jean Campbell had left upon him.

He stood up and walked towards an alcove. From a drinks tray, he took two glasses and poured whisky into both from a decanter. More fingers of the spirit than was usual. He handed Dr Wilson a glass and sat down again. The doctor's hand trembled as he accepted it.

They sat in silence for some moments.

Charles spoke first. 'I want her gone from here. Can you arrange that?'

Dr Wilson looked confused. 'Arrange what, exactly?'

'A way to shut her up, Wilson,' Charles replied. 'The genie is out of the bottle. There's no controlling her. The stupid bitch is a liability.'

The old doctor stared at a patch of carpet. He looked bewildered, as if he were wrestling with a conscience so ineffectual that he could find no courage to stand up to this man.

'I won't do anything illegal, Charles.'

Charles began to laugh. 'For fuck's sake, Wilson. Did you think I was asking you to do away with her?'

'To be honest, nothing would surprise me,' Dr Wilson replied. 'It's not exactly a common or garden situation we're embroiled in here.'

Charles glowered. 'Listen to me, you old soak. Be under no illusion. If I could get away with murdering her, I'd do it in a heartbeat. I'd do it myself with no help from you. I'd fucking enjoy it and all.'

'You don't mean that, Charles. She's your wife, for pity's sake.'

Charles looked at the doctor as if he were an imbecile.

'Of course I mean it. Euphemia has proven herself to be an utter impediment to my future. She has no gratitude for what I've done for her. I procured her a healthy baby to cover up for her female failings but, instead of thanking me and looking after the child, she decided to dash its brains out on a hearthstone.'

Charles's indignation was such that it threatened to overcome him.

'Now, when I've spent hours putting myself in danger to cover up the mess she's made, all she's able to do is rant and rave and claw at herself.'

Dr Wilson held out his hands in a placatory manner, as much to keep away the surfeit of emotion as to mollify McDougall.

'I don't think her mind is sound, Charles. Perhaps some fellow feeling might prove helpful under the circumstances?'

'Any feeling I had for her is long gone. That woman upstairs is nothing to do with me anymore. I want her away from the house any way I can manage. I never want to see her again. She's obviously insane. I am relying on you to find a place for her to go.'

'An asylum?'

'Yes,' Charles said. 'Why not? Somewhere that they'll lock her up and shut her up. If they feed her on bread and water, so much the better.'

Dr Wilson shook his head. 'I can't send Euphemia to a madhouse. Surely to God you wouldn't see your wife carted off to Clyde Street, Charles. It's like a vision of Hell down there – full of filthy lunatics – and it regularly gets consumed by flooding from the river. It's not sanitary. It's certainly not a place for a respectable woman, no matter what she's done.'

Charles drummed his fingers against his glass.

'What about this new building in Parliamentary Row? The one they've built to Stark's design?'

Dr Wilson shook his head. 'It's not complete yet. Anyway, if we're talking about a public asylum, no matter how progressive it is, the parish have to rubber-stamp any application on behalf of a patient. I'm not sure you'd want another doctor to examine Euphemia to see if they agree with my diagnosis. She might tell them what she's done, and they might not think it's the jabber of a lunatic. They might well believe her.'

Charles looked angry. 'I'm not looking for help from the parish. What do you take me for? I can pay for her place.'

'It doesn't matter,' said Dr Wilson. 'Even private patients have to be certified and examined by the authorities. My say-so isn't enough.'

'For fuck's sake. There must be another way. Surely to God when I've got the money to pay for it.'

Dr Wilson sighed. 'There are private houses where they take in cases. That might be an option.'

'What do you mean, private?' Charles asked.

'Independent of the authorities,' replied the doctor. 'I know of a couple of large country houses run as asylums in Stirlingshire and Lanarkshire. There are also a few smaller concerns. Houses that look after a few patients, sometimes only one or two.'

Charles considered this for a moment. 'Who are they run by?'

'Some are managed by retired medical practitioners, some ex-attendants from the big hospitals,' Dr Wilson said. 'They look like ordinary villas from the outside. It's a more discreet route than the municipal asylums.'

'But don't you still need two doctors to agree?'

274

Dr Wilson pursed his lips. 'Strictly speaking, yes, but there are places that can find doctors who are willing to provide a second opinion on the patient for a small consideration.'

Charles snorted with laughter. 'And you'd know this how, Wilson? Are you, by any chance, one of these tame doctors?'

Dr Wilson affected to ignore this comment and carried on.

'There's a place near Torrance that might suit your needs.'

~

When they had finished their whiskies, the two men went upstairs to Euphemia's bedroom and unlocked the door. She was sleeping. After Dr Wilson had subdued her, he had summoned the maid.

Martha had adjusted Euphemia's nightclothes and tucked her up beneath the sheets, covers and eiderdown. The obvious tenderness that the girl had shown her mistress worried at Dr Wilson's conscience.

Charles, for his part, was oblivious. He had a problem and a possible solution that he needed to learn more about. He was beginning to enjoy his strategising. He looked at his wife lying on the bed. Her hair smoothed into her broderie-trimmed nightcap; the blue ribbon tied neatly under her chin. Charles had to decide how best to move her. She might as well have been a consignment of herring from the North Sea or Lanarkshire coal heading to Oban. It was all one to him.

'How soon can we get her to this house at Torrance?' he asked the doctor.

'I'll send word to them tomorrow and stress the urgency

of the request. If they are willing to take her, it shouldn't be more than a couple of days.'

'And this place, is it secure?'

Dr Wilson nodded.

'She won't be allowed to wander?' Charles asked. 'They can restrain her if needs be?

'Yes.'

Charles felt his prick harden. He imagined Euphemia shackled to a bed and he felt almost sorry that he wouldn't be there to enjoy it.

52

∾ Tuesday, 18 March 1817:
The High Court, Edinburgh ∾

Robert breakfasted early and made his way back to the High Court in a torrent of rain.

Once inside and divested of his soaking greatcoat, he stood awkwardly in the foyer waiting, as instructed, for Archibald Gibson to appear. A huge mirror took up much of the wall facing him and Robert caught sight of his reflection. He rifled his fingers through his hair, trying to coax it into presentability, and bent down to brush off the smuts that had gathered at the sides of his shoes. The foyer was carpeted with a long oriental rug. Robert stared at a patch of exposed warp and weft where the pile had completely worn away. He guessed Jean would be in the cells below. No doubt Sibbald would have walked her the short distance from the Tolbooth.

Presently, Gibson arrived, and the two men climbed the stairs to the courtroom, empty apart from some junior clerks organising papers at tables and a couple of ushers officiating at the doors. Robert took a seat that had been provided for him directly under the witness box.

The court filled quickly, Jean was brought in and Succoth took his seat. After some preliminaries, His Lordship turned to the defence counsel. Mr McNeil opened the case for the defence by returning first to the question of the accused's deafness.

'Gentlemen,' he began, 'you are charged with deciding the guilt or innocence of a deaf and dumb woman. While the panel may have been judged fit to plead and thus fit to face the consequences of her actions, it is my assertion that her inability to hear is something that merits further consideration—'

Succoth interrupted the defence counsel by clearing his throat. 'In what way does it merit further consideration, Mr McNeil? I'll need to insist you be specific regarding this matter. The court has made a judgement about the panel's suitability for trial and provided an interpreter. I am disinclined to waste any more time discussing abstract theories of deafness.'

'Forgive me, my Lord, these are not simply theories,' said McNeil. 'What I would like to impart to the jury is information about the practicalities of being deaf and the impact that the condition has on the lives of the afflicted. I believe that it is important to understand the panel's experience in order to decide if what she has done was a deliberate act or an accident of circumstance.'

Succoth considered this for a second. 'Very well, but keep it within the confines of what is necessary, Mr McNeil. I don't want the business of the court winding down sundry or esoteric paths.'

McNeil made a little nod of acknowledgement and outlined his intention to call back to the court the three experts who had judged Jean's fitness to plead, the panel herself and a character witness to attest to her previous conduct in Glasgow.

An usher took a piece of paper proffered by one of McNeil's assistants and went out into the foyer to call the witness to the courtroom. Edwin Browne took the stand once again.

'Dr Browne, can you explain the reasons why some

unfortunates are born deaf and dumb and how it affects the body and mind of those who suffer from it?'

Robert watched as Dr Browne attempted to smooth his unruly whiskers. 'Certainly,' the doctor began. 'From a medical point of view, we can explain something of the origins of deafness. It is a result of the component parts of the ear being in a damaged or diseased state. In the majority of cases that I have had experience of, this means that the auditory nerve has suffered some break in its connection to the brain. In a few individuals, deafness may be caused by the diseased state of the brain itself. However, there remains much investigation to be done in terms of the study of the complexities of the inner workings of the ear as well as of those who are affected by deafness.'

McNeil made a great show of pondering this testimony and regarded the jury with a look that suggested they should give Dr Browne's statements the same serious amount of consideration as he was.

'This affliction. What are the current theories as to its cause?' asked McNeil.

'There are many schools of thought; not all of them in agreement with each other,' Dr Browne said. 'It is the opinion of some that deafness is hereditary but, looking at the facts, in families where there are one or more deaf children, they are no more likely to have had antecedents with a similar defect than a child who is able to hear. Others believe that the occurrence of deafness is altogether accidental and is likely to be caused by the position or state of the foetus in the mother's womb. Yet another theory is that the condition is owing to some defect of mind of the mother during the period of gestation. Another school of thought posits that there is something peculiar about the head shape of deaf and dumb people; being longer and having indentation at the sides.'

'What is your own view, doctor?' asked McNeil.

'I am inclined to believe that deafness happens in utero, that is, during the period of gestation. As to the exact cause, that is still a mystery. It is perfectly common for a healthy mother who has had no problems during pregnancy to give birth to a deaf baby.'

'And are you able to tell us what percentage of the population are deaf and dumb?' McNeil asked.

Dr Browne shook his head.

'Not with any degree of accuracy, I'm afraid. We believe there are several hundreds of people in Scotland who were born deaf and, as a consequence of that accident of birth, are also dumb. A comprehensive survey on the state of the poor has recently been proposed by parliament that, if and when completed, should give us a more accurate picture. I'm afraid, however, that is of no help to the court today.'

'Are the deaf completely unable to hear, just as the blind cannot see?' McNeil asked.

'There are variations in the extent of a deaf and dumb person's hearing, just as there are variations in the level of blindness. The tests that we use are designed to estab-lish if someone does not have enough hearing to process information through the ear and develop language by imitation.'

'But deaf people have been taught to speak, is that right?'

'Yes, many who are born deaf and dumb acquire the skills to pronounce words but the sound they make is abrasive to our ears since they are unable to regulate tone.'

'So, if the deaf can acquire these skills, despite their lack of the sense needed to develop speech, their intellect cannot be in question.'

Dr Browne agreed. 'Their intellect varies in exactly the same way it does in the rest of the population.'

'In that respect, the deaf and dumb are the same as you or me, doctor?'

'It is my opinion that they are.'

Robert glanced across at the jury. The two rows of gentlemen had concentrated hard on what Edwin Browne had had to say. Robert thought it unlikely that any of them knew anyone who was deaf, except perhaps those unfortunate enough to be forced to throw themselves on the mercy of the local parish or beg for alms in the closes of the old town. While Dr Browne's testimony was well-evidenced and fair, Robert couldn't help but suspect that Jean Campbell was no more than a curio to these men, something already destined to become a prurient dinner-table anecdote in the future.

The next witness was called. It was to be the panel herself. Robert took a breath and gathered himself as Jean was led to the witness box. She stood waiting while Succoth instructed Robert to interpret for her once again. There was some momentary confusion as McNeil began his questioning, then halted as he realised that he was directing his questions to someone who couldn't hear them and then looked to Robert for clarification.

'Should I speak to yourself or to the panel?' the lawyer asked.

'Perhaps to the court in general, sir?' suggested Robert. 'I can relay your words to Miss Campbell and convey her answers in the direction of both yourself and the jury?'

'Very well, Mr Kinniburgh.'

McNeil raised his hands to straighten his robes and outlined his first question.

'Yesterday, when she was sworn in, the panel told the court that she was not guilty of the charge of murder of a child. However, she did not deny that a child fell into the River Clyde from the Old Bridge and, further, that it fell as a result of her loosening her grip on it. Mr Kinniburgh, can you ask the panel whose child it was?'

Robert turned to Jean and signed, *Was it your baby that fell from the bridge?*

Yes. It was my wee boy.

When this was relayed, McNeil followed it up by asking how old the baby was.

Just over three weeks, Jean signed.

'Did you mean to throw it into the river?'

Jean shook her head.

'How did it come to fall?'

Robert splayed his fingers and followed their trajectory, as if watching Jean's baby disappear into the water.

I was very tired. I stopped to wrap him tighter inside my shawl. I lost hold of him.

'Was your baby dead or alive when it fell?' asked McNeil.

There was a hush in the room as Robert signed the question to her. Most, if not all, of those present knew nothing of sign language, but watched his hands intently and could not have failed to notice the adverse connotation of fingers pointed downwards in contrast to the more favourable circle skimming over Robert's heart.

All eyes turned to Jean. With both hands in front of her, she pointed her index and middle fingers sharply towards the grave.

'How did the baby die?' McNeil asked.

The mistress of the house where I was living. She killed him.

McNeil looked astonished.

Succoth raised his hand to halt proceedings. 'No more of this havering. Does she have evidence to back up that claim, Kinniburgh?'

'She does not, Your Lordship.'

'Then we cannot hear it. The woman is quite naturally

disturbed by the death of her child. Is this a fantasy of her own making to assuage a mother's guilt?'

Robert looked at Succoth. As far as His Lordship was concerned, they were here to decide if Jean's baby had fallen by accident or design from the Old Bridge. Up until now, everything that had been evidenced could be explained in the context of a distraught mother carrying the body of her dead child to somewhere safe, a church or the city hospital or the police office. The jury might have sympathy for her plight, but they would take their cues from Succoth. If His Lordship took a dim view of Jean's testimony, the members of the jury might well follow suit.

'Perhaps, Your Lordship.' Robert dropped his glance to the floor. He could not bear to look at Jean.

'Quite so,' said Succoth. 'The first month of life is a precarious time. So many infants are not viable. They are brought into the world out of godless union; perhaps it is a kindness.'

~

As it was nearing the middle of the day, Succoth called for an hour's break in proceedings to allow people to relieve themselves and get something to eat and drink.

When the court reconvened, McNeil called Robert to the stand.

'Mr Kinniburgh, you are concerned in the education of deaf children. In your experience, are they as intelligent and receptive to instruction as those who can hear?'

'In terms of intelligence, I would say so. However, they require a different type of instruction than hearing children and the process of imparting knowledge often takes longer.'

'Why is that?'

'I teach approximately fifty pupils in the Deaf and Dumb

Institution. They are of different ages, come from a variety of backgrounds and have a wide range of educational experiences by the time they arrive at my school. Some of them have been encouraged and instructed by their families and communities. Others have been given little stimulation or support. In addition, they have not grown up in the society of the deaf and dumb, so they have not had the opportunity to communicate with other people with the same condition. This lack of cohesion means that the normal system of educating by rote and to a large cohort of pupils at once is not feasible.'

'And how do you deal with these problems?' asked McNeil.

'We teach in small groups and encourage the older pupils to work with younger ones, to share knowledge and skills.'

'And do you use signs?'

'We teach the children to read and write English in order that they can acquire information from books. However, signing is the preferred way for the deaf and dumb to communicate between themselves, so it is often easier to explain a concept by signs.'

'Does using this sign language hinder the deaf and dumb in their ability to become useful members of society?' McNeil asked. 'What is the benefit of signing if it is merely a different version of the written language?'

'I'm not entirely sure, sir,' Robert replied. 'I only know that using signs comes naturally to all the deaf children that are in my care and that forcing them not to use this natural method of communication is often the cause of much distress to them. In any event, I believe that the language of signs is not merely a mimicking of our own language. I think it has its own rules and is more suited to those who can see but who cannot hear.'

At this point, McNeil, who had been standing near the

witness box, approached the area where the jury were seated. He leant against the wooden barrier that separated them from the other spectators and glanced at them, conspiratorially. 'But it is a crude and basic language, it has some savagery in its mode of communication compared to ours, does it not?'

Robert was shocked. He did not wish to be included in McNeil's definition of 'ours'. 'No,' he replied, vehemently. 'I believe it often looks so to those who do not have sign language, but that is due to others' lack of understanding rather than any defect in the language itself.'

'You wouldn't agree with the speculation that the deaf and dumb are more aggressive than the rest of us?'

'Not at all.'

McNeil smiled indulgently at Robert, as if he somehow knew better than the teacher. 'Thank you, Mr Kinniburgh.'

Next, McNeil recalled Jeremiah Pringle and continued his line of questioning.

'Professor Pringle, you are an expert in the field of moral philosophy. Would you agree with Mr Kinniburgh, that the deaf and dumb are not necessarily more aggressive than those with the gift of hearing?'

'Yes, I would. In fact, I'd go even further and say that the visual and kinetic elements of their signing language notwithstanding, they are gentler than the hearing population in almost all respects.'

'In what way?' asked McNeil, incredulously.

'In the sense that they have long been considered to be more naturally connected to the world and more sensitive to its workings.'

'Can you explain more of what you mean, Professor?'

'Reaching back into time, we see many instances where the common people of this country and of other places on the world ascribe qualities to the deaf and dumb that could be considered spiritual or mystical or psychic in some way. Some have been said to foretell coming events. For instance, there are tales of deaf and dumb people seeing into the future and warning of the failure of crops or a sudden change of sea conditions.'

McNeil blinked. 'Surely this is merely ignorance and superstition?'

Pringle gave a thin smile. 'It is possible that these stories can be attributed to backward and uninformed minds. However, it is also possible that the deaf and dumb possess an unusual degree of innate intelligence that, unhindered by the noise of our modern world, operates on a more compassionate and sympathetic level than it does for the rest of us.'

'You mentioned earlier that you believed Jean Campbell capable of finer feelings than other people. On what evidence do you base this?'

'I have studied many people who have mental and physical afflictions. The deaf and dumb that I have observed appear to be acutely aware of their surroundings and are often badly affected by aggression or violence. I believe this to be because they do not hear the language of ruffianism that is so prevalent now.'

Succoth interjected. 'Exactly how is this line of questioning relevant to the charge of murder that this woman faces?'

'I apologise, my Lord,' McNeil said obsequiously. 'I will attempt to clarify.'

Returning to Pringle, the defence counsel continued, 'This increase in sensitivity that you've mentioned, could it make Jean Campbell more or less likely to commit a crime?'

'Oh, much less likely. The idea of causing pain to another person – especially her own child – would be anathema to her. She would find the concept abhorrent.'

McNeil nodded. 'Could this explain her extreme distress on being arrested and taken to the police office in Glasgow?'

'I very much believe it could, yes.'

When Pringle had exited the witness box, Angus Buchanan took the stand in his full clergyman's regalia. He attested to Jean's good character and fervently rejected the image of her as one of the undesirables that hung around the Saltmarket, drinking and hooring. Robert was impressed by his composure. Angus spoke knowledgeably and eloquently, outlining Jean's stable working life and family support before she had fallen in with an Irishman.

Robert hoped it was enough.

53

∼ Monday, 24 February 1817:
Partickhill Road, Glasgow ∼

The front door slammed and made Martha jump. She and Ina glanced at each other in silent recognition that the master had returned home. They both stood stock still for a moment until Ina rubbed her hands on her apron and unfastened it. She went out to the back green and shook it out, a cloud of dirt and stoor bursting into the air. Martha resisted the temptation to go outside too. Her heart was beating nineteen to the dozen at the thought that Mr McDougall might come down to the kitchen and find her there.

All afternoon, they had moved through the house like ghosts, doing the bidding of Dr Wilson as he watched over Euphemia. All three of them, the maid, the cook and the doctor, waited in a kind of limbo, to see what might happen next. None of them could conceive of the situation getting worse but neither could they imagine it getting any better.

As soon as Mr McDougall had left in pursuit of Jean, Ina had sent Martha down the brae to fetch the doctor. The mistress could not be reasoned with and the old woman was neither equipped nor willing to take charge of the situation on her own. Martha had asked if she shouldn't go for a policeman instead – she could run down to the inn at the bottom of the hill and raise the alarm. Ina shook her head. Someone else could make those kinds of decisions. The less the two of them were involved, the better.

The last thing that a young lassie like Martha needed was to be dragged to a police office to give a statement. And Ina didn't trust either of the McDougalls. Especially the master. Ina didn't trust that one at all. He was the type that would turn on you, make up a story to cover up his own sins and implicate others. Ina Drysdale counselled Martha to caw canny and bide her time.

~

When the pair of them walked into the drawing room, they found Mr McDougall slumped in a chair. It was unheard of for servants not to knock and wait for permission to enter a room. Charles looked up, more startled than angry at their lack of propriety.

Martha wished that the ground would open and swallow her whole. Ina, on the other hand, didn't flinch. If the old woman was intimidated in this environment, she certainly wasn't showing it. Ina was in high dudgeon. As Martha had trailed up the stairs in her wake, Ina had told her not to worry, there was no reason for either of them to be frightened of this jumped-up nobody. She would speak plainly to him and, if Charles McDougall touched a hair on their heads, there would be a mob of Partick men at his door in no time. He might act the big man on the surface but, deep down, Charles McDougall knew that Ina was wise to him, that she knew a coward when she met one.

They had been embroiled in a subtle game of wits for the last few years. Both dancing around each other, Ina deferring to him and he playing the role of the master. Mr McDougall had taken great care of the way that he issued instructions to her, being sure not to overstep the mark. Ina was sharp as a whip and Charles felt that, beneath her deference, she could see right through to his miserable soul. Yet, if someone had asked Charles for his opinion of his housekeeper, he would have affected utter disinterest about the old woman from the dockside cottages who prepared his meals and kept his pantry stocked.

Euphemia, on the other hand, knew instinctively how to deal with servants. She had been brought up to it and seemed to negotiate any situation with ease. His wife behaved in an altogether neutral way with Mrs Drysdale, something that Charles could never hope to achieve. Instead, he came across as boorish and entitled, which the cook accurately read as showing a lack of self-confidence, an inadequate substitute for breeding.

Martha watched as Ina stood before him, quiet and self-contained. A steely gaze in her eye; full of determination. Her lack of obvious emotion was at odds with the master's own demeanour. His hair was unruly, his breathing still ragged with panic, his collar torn and flapping loose from his jacket.

'Did you want something, Mrs Drysdale?'

'Aye, sir.' Ina looked at him with disdain. 'I came to tell you that the doctor's upstairs. He's made the mistress calm, sir. We were worried she'd harm herself.'

'Heaven forfend,' Charles muttered.

Ina pretended not to hear him.

'I just came to tell you I'll be off now, sir, if that's acceptable?'

Martha wondered at the sarcasm implicit in Ina's tone but the master either didn't notice or was pretending not to have heard.

'Yes, Mrs Drysdale. Thank you for staying on while I was called away.'

Ina said nothing and Mr McDougall waited for her to take her leave. He obviously couldn't wait to see the back of her.

'I'm afraid I won't be here tomorrow, sir.'

Martha did a quick mental calculation. It was Tuesday tomorrow. Surely Ina's day off was a Thursday? Mr McDougall seemed to be doing the same. Perhaps wondering if the cook had agreed something with Euphemia that he knew nothing about.

'Or any day after that, sir.'

'I beg your pardon, Mrs Drysdale?' he said. 'Are you asking to leave my employ? We agreed on a month's notice, did we not?' The master looked confused. Was there something wrong with the old woman, some kind of sickness that he wasn't supposed to know about? 'Have you spoken to my wife about this?'

Ina snorted. 'No. I doubt she would have listened, even if I had. She's that doped up, she disnae know up from down.'

The sirs and the pretence of submission had disappeared now. A wave of dread enveloped Martha and her knees began to tremble.

Ina took a deep breath and straightened her back. She was at least a foot smaller than the master but, at that moment, it didn't seem to be a disadvantage.

'I won't be giving any notice, Mr McDougall. I don't think that will be necessary under the present circumstances.'

There was a long silence.

'Do you intend to tell anyone what occurred here today?' Mr McDougall swallowed. 'The police, for example.'

Ina shrugged and asked, 'Is Jean Campbell alive?'

'Yes,' said Mr McDougall.

Ina considered his dishevelled appearance. 'Not for want of trying on your part, though?'

The master reached into his jacket for his pocketbook. 'I have money,' he said. He took out a bundle of notes and handed them to Ina. She extended her hand slowly and took them, tucked them inside her skirt pocket.

Mr McDougall regarded her. 'I expect your silence on this matter.'

'Oh, you'll have it. What else would I do?' Ina asked. 'Go to the police? Tell them you and your wife killed a helpless infant? You'd likely deny all knowledge or blame poor Jean. What would be the point?'

'None at all,' said Mr McDougall. 'There's no need for anyone else to get hurt.'

His tone was conciliatory, but Martha sensed an implicit threat.

Ina paused for a second. Martha hoped this was them finished and she would be able to leave the room, but Ina carried on as if she had decided that she had nothing to lose.

'You listen to me for a minute, McDougall,' she began. 'The only reason I'm not going to the police is that, despite what she's done, I feel nothing but pity for that poor creature that's married to you. Make no mistake, if I thought you were the one that would hang for the wee one's death, I'd have been down to the Partick police office like a shot.'

Ina put her arm around Martha and ushered her to the door. As they were leaving, she looked back at the master.

'And mind you watch your step with this wee lassie while she's still under your roof. I'll be speaking to her faither. I'll tell him she'd be better off out of here. He'll be up to collect her as soon as he's able.'

Ina reached out for the doorknob. From nothing more than force of habit she backed out and shut the door quietly behind her.

54

~ Tuesday, 18 March 1817:
The High Court, Edinburgh ~

It was getting late. The high windows of the courtroom no longer admitted any light. Orderlies shuffled quietly, undertaking the practicalities involved in shifting operations from day to night. Candles in sconces around the perimeter of the room were lit and a scattering of oil lamps were carried in and afforded to those who were required to read from official documents and record the proceedings.

Succoth peered into the gloom and first asked McCormack to summarise the prosecution's case and then invited McNeil to advocate on behalf of the prisoner. McCormack adopted a bullish aspect and pushed for a guilty verdict, citing the incontrovertible testimony of those on the bridge. Surely, the prosecution counsel suggested, these witnesses could not all have been mistaken. They had seen a small body wrapped against the cold, they had witnessed something meet with the water of the Clyde, they had heard a scream ring out into the dark of a winter's evening. Yes, of course it had been gloomy and poorly lit, it was a scene wreathed in fog and wrought with confusion. But these witnesses were local folk, hard-working people who had no reason to lie to the court. In his view, it was likely that Jean Campbell had thrown her baby's body into the river and that she had done it intentionally, perhaps to conceal the already dead infant, who could say?

McNeil, for his part, appealed to the jury for sympathy

for this poor woman who was as much victim as perpetrator and asked them to find her not guilty. He acknowledged the testimony of the witnesses and agreed that there was no reason for the jury to suspect they were telling anything but the truth of what they had observed. However, McNeil argued, there was no proof that Jean Campbell had allowed her baby to fall from the bridge. Eyes and ears, even the keenest, played tricks on people in the dark. And, as Lord Succoth had pointed out, newly born babies suffered huge rates of mortality – why would this woman have needed to conceal the fact of yet another infant's death? The jury had heard testimony from the most learned and upright of gentlemen attesting to her previously good character and her distress and confusion as to the turn of events and her current circumstances. Is it not more likely that she is an innocent caught up in a series of unfortunate misunderstandings?

Robert watched the members of the jury as the two sides made their appeals. Some leant forward, deep in concentration, listening to what the two counsels had to say, brows furrowed as they contemplated the difficulty of their task. There were two sides to every story, they seemed to be thinking, but what if neither was sufficiently compelling to make you throw your lot in with it?

Finally, Lord Succoth addressed the jury. He reiterated the detail of their task.

'Gentlemen, a summary of their arguments has been put forward from both prosecution and defence counsels. You have heard first-hand testimony from eyewitnesses to the events on the Old Bridge in Glasgow on the twenty-fourth of February. You have listened patiently as experts have told us of the present condition of the deaf and dumb and the possible impact that affliction might have had on the accused. As to Jean Campbell herself, a respected clergyman has furnished you with a heartfelt description of her character and reputation, refuting any assumptions made as to her sex and her class.'

Succoth paused for a second, taking a sip from a glass of water.

'On the other hand, a baby has died. The lady has told us this herself. However, she cannot or will not provide an explanation for this death to the court. This state of affairs is not merely frustrating, it is potentially criminal, and you must weigh up what you have been told by all parties before you come to a decision in this case.'

Succoth reached for his glass and took a sip of water.

'You must now decide whether the evidence put before you allows you to forward a verdict of guilty or not guilty. If it does not, you may return a verdict of not proven. The key question that should guide you is this; was the child's fatal fall a result of malice or of accident?'

Robert looked over at Jean. She sat very still, her drab clothing merging into her surroundings. Only her pale skin stood out, like an alabaster statue in the corner of a country church.

He sighed. They were like puppets in a shadow-play, he and she, brought out to perform and then packed away with no chance to determine how their story ended.

'If you can come to a decision quickly,' Succoth continued, 'you may give it now. If you wish to request more time to discuss your verdict, you should make that known to the clerk.'

The fifteen men who made up the jury were sitting over two rows of benches directly facing the witness box. A clerk, who had been perched by the side of this assembly, stood up and consulted with one of their number; a tall, patrician man with a thoughtful expression, who Robert assumed had been chosen as their spokesman.

The tall man turned to his fellows and they gathered together in mumbled conversation. Robert supposed they were deliberating, either about the verdict itself or whether to ask to be excused to debate the case.

Then, quite suddenly, and without quitting their box, they returned a verdict of not proven.

Tears pricked at Robert's eyes and he tried to steady their flow. Jean still sat quietly, utterly oblivious to her fate. He longed to stand up and celebrate, could feel a grin spreading on his face but he took a deep breath and collected himself.

Lord Succoth thanked the jury.

'The prisoner is dismissed from the bar,' he declared. Then caught himself as he seemed to realise that Jean couldn't understand him. 'Mr Kinniburgh, can you lend us your assistance once more?'

Robert was up on his feet in an instant. He was acutely aware of Jean, still standing in the dock, unaware of what was going on even though, when all was said and done, it affected her and her alone.

'I would be delighted to, my Lord.'

It was only when he faced Jean that he realised he had no idea how to sign the verdict. He had no handshape for *not proven*. In the end, he settled on something that would make sense to Jean. *You are free.* He splayed his hands in a burst in front of his chest, fingers outstretched and expansive.

Jean looked at him curiously for a moment and responded, *Free? I can go home?*

Robert nodded and grinned at her, his heart hammering with relief in his chest. He wanted to embrace her, but propriety held him back. Instead, Angus rushed forward and took her from her seat. They hugged each other and Robert retreated.

Succoth called the court to order again. His Lordship

expressed a wish that some attention be given to the instruction of Jean Campbell in future; it would be wholly wrong, in his opinion, for her to fall back into the straits in which she had found herself. Perhaps the Institution of the Deaf and Dumb could help her in some way?

Robert hadn't anticipated this turn of events.

'I'm sorry, my Lord, but Miss Campbell is beyond the age of being entered into my institution.'

'In that case, Mr Kinniburgh, would you be willing to ensure that she is taken home to her native place in Islay?'

'Yes, my Lord, if that is the wish of the court.'

Then, by desire of Lord Succoth, he was requested to communicate this to Jean herself, which he did; the prisoner nodded her understanding, made her obeisance to the court and retired.

55

~ Friday, 21 March 1817:
Saltmarket, Glasgow ~

It was raining heavily as Robert, Angus and David walked down the Saltmarket. They were headed in the direction of Jim Donnelly's lodgings in Taylor's Close.

Water tumbled down makeshift gutters and swept across their path and the three men had to pick their way across on some dislodged paving stones that stood proud from the surface of the street. It was like using stepping stones to cross a fast-flowing river, only a deal less bucolic.

Robert had disembarked from the Edinburgh stage no more than a quarter of an hour earlier and found the minister and his son waiting for him at the Tontine. Angus pressed upon him the news that there was no time to lose if they wanted to catch up with the Irishman, so Robert left his baggage at the entrance to the hotel with word that he would return without delay.

As they headed away from the wide sweep of Argyle Street, Angus explained the circumstances behind the brief letter he had sent to Robert, urging him to travel to Glasgow.

'As you know, I made my way back home on the night stage immediately after the trial,' said Angus. 'Once I knew that they would release Jean into my care, I determined to get us both back as soon as I could and let her friends and family know that a not proven verdict had been returned.

I knew that they would all be greatly relieved to know the outcome.'

'Where is Jean now?' asked Robert.

Angus smiled. 'She's at the manse, with Catriona. Being fed and watered and rested. I reasoned that I could await your instructions as to Jean's journey back to Islay and, positioned in Glasgow, I could make any practical arrangements that you deemed necessary.'

Angus took a breath as they turned into the Briggait.

'When I got home, the day had barely begun, but Catriona was already up and waiting for me,' Angus explained. 'Do you remember leaving your name with the family who live across the landing from Donnelly?'

'Of course,' said Robert. 'I spoke to a young girl and her mother.'

'Well,' Angus continued, 'it transpired that the woman had called at the Tontine to tell you that Jim Donnelly had returned to his lodgings. He was only going to be back in Glasgow briefly, as he intended re-joining the team working on the canals in a matter of days. This must have been the same day that Jean's trial was being heard.'

'So how on earth did your wife hear this news?' asked Robert.

'The staff at the Tontine told the woman that I had been helping you in your work and they gave her the name of our church. Thank goodness Donnelly's neighbour thought her information was sufficiently important to seek us out.'

Robert sighed. 'It would have been better if we'd found him before the trial.'

'Are you sure about that?' asked Angus. 'What would it have achieved? Donnelly would only have been able to confirm part of Jean's story about the McDougalls. He had no idea about what happened to the baby. In fact, any evidence he gave would have placed Jean in the McDougall household with the express purpose of selling her baby to them and that might have made the jury more likely to return a guilty verdict.'

Robert conceded that Angus had a point.

'But,' Angus continued, 'Donnelly might well know where to look for Jean's son, so we need to find him before Jean makes the journey to Islay.'

'Have you booked passage for both of them; Jean and Sandy?' Robert asked Angus.

'I have, and yourself. I'm still hopeful that we can find the boy, but we have very little time.'

When the three men reached Taylor's Close, Robert located the entrance to the stairwell once again and led the way up the stairs. The door to Donnelly's lodging was shut and no one answered when Robert knocked. They stood for a few seconds, unsure of what to do next, but then David reached down and turned the handle. It wasn't locked. Gingerly, they looked inside.

The room was small and sparsely furnished. Donnelly was sitting on the bed. He was shirtless, wearing only a pair of woollen trousers, braces trailed on the sheets. The Irishman didn't seem to have noticed that strangers had entered his dwelling place. Slumped as he was, he looked a powerful man; a lifetime of labouring had left its mark in muscle and sinew.

'Mr Donnelly,' Robert said, 'we're here with news of Jean. May we talk with you a while?'

Donnelly spun round.

'Is she to hang?' he asked.

Robert shook his head. 'No. She's been released. The court found the case not proven.'

Donnelly looked confused. 'Does that mean they know she's not guilty?'

'It means that the facts don't add up and they couldn't decide either way,' said Angus. 'No matter, it's all one. It means they have let her out.'

Donnelly seemed to deflate again.

'Are you alright there, Mr Donnelly?' Angus asked him.

The Irishman turned and stared at them, as if seeing them for the first time.

'I'm glad Jean's not to hang,' he said. 'I don't believe she would have harmed our child.'

'But you ran away, nonetheless,' said Robert.

Jim stood up abruptly and they all took a step backwards, unsure of what the man might do next. Robert was glad that they had brought David with them. He was younger and fitter than Angus and Robert himself was no fighter.

Angus approached Donnelly, reaching an arm out to clasp his shoulder. Perhaps it was this kind gesture or the sight of Angus's clerical collar, but the wind seemed to suddenly be taken out of Jim's sails.

'What was I supposed to do? It was me got her into trouble in the first place,' he said defensively.

'You could have stayed and spoken up for her,' Robert said. 'You could have told the police that she had been staying with the McDougalls. Then they might have discovered what really happened. There could have been evidence to prove what they had done.'

'What do you mean, what they had done?' Donnelly asked. 'Who are you talking about – the McDougalls?'

'I can tell you about it, if you want?'

Jim nodded.

There was a stool by the window. Robert pulled it over nearer Donnelly and began to explain.

～

Donnelly balled the dirty bed sheets in his fists and stared at Robert.

'Are you sure?' he asked.

'I'm sure.'

'I'll fucking kill both of them, in that case.'

Robert shook his head. 'I'd like to see you try. McDougall's absconded and he's shut his wife up in a madhouse. I don't see them answering for what they've done.'

'They can't get away with this,' Donnelly roared.

Robert looked at him like he was a child. 'Of course they can, Mr Donnelly. There's no evidence to tie them to the crime. Even if there was, it's too late. Jean has been tried for the murder. As far as the law is concerned, all of this talk of the McDougalls is just irrelevant rumour and conjecture.'

Angus stepped forward. 'You can still help Jean, Mr Donnelly.'

'How?'

'We are trying to find her son, Sandy. She wants to see him but, more pressingly, is desperate to ensure that he is safe. No one knows what became of him after the evening that Jean was arrested.'

'I saw him took,' said Jim. 'Outside the police office. A man had a hold of him.'

Angus looked at him askance. 'But I've been to the local poorhouse. I spoke to the superintendent. There's no Sandy Campbell there.'

Robert thought for a moment.

'Perhaps we should take another look, Angus?'

56

∼ Saturday, 22 March 1817:
Bardowie, Stirlingshire ∼

The Dr Wilson that Martha had mentioned to Robert turned out to be well-known in the city and had furnished Angus with an address for the asylum. It was some miles north of the city and was reached by the Balmore Road. The doctor had claimed ignorance as to the whereabouts of Charles McDougall, but he had imparted some information about the financial arrangements lately agreed between McDougall and his father-in-law.

Angus had managed to find Robert a lift from a carter who was going as far as Lambhill Stables on the canal. The carter was on his way to fetch some coal from a barge and bring it back to Glasgow. Robert sat alongside him in the front of the cart, both of them passing the time in talking and smoking as they trundled along. First over the paved streets that led up to Cowcaddens, and then on to unmade paths and eventually country roads fringed with trees coming into bud.

When the carter halted at Lambhill, Robert climbed down and continued the last couple of miles of his journey on foot. Houses were strung like beads along the narrow road but even these thinned out after a short time and Robert found himself winding through open farmland on either side.

As he breasted a slope, he sat down under a tree and ate the lunch of bread and dripping that Mrs Buchanan had given to Angus for him. A stream flowed past at the bottom of the brae and, after he finished eating, Robert edged down though tussocks of grass still browned by the winter. He bent down and filled his flask up with cold water, guessing by the geography that the stream was either the Allander Water or the early stages of the River Kelvin. He took a long drink and then refilled the flask to make sure he had enough to complete his travels. The fields around him lay scrubbed and barren, awaiting a new year's planting.

Soon, Robert came to a junction where there was a meeting of roads. The carter had directed him to turn right along a road opposite the tollhouse, so Robert did as he had been bidden. On his left-hand side, the fields swept down to a small loch that lay empty and dark and still. As he approached a barn, he saw a young man clearing piles of dirty straw from its entrance.

'Could you tell me if I'm on the right road for Blackfaulds House?'

The young man stopped his work and walked over to where Robert stood at the gate to the road.

'Aye, you've not far to go.' He pointed to a bend in the road. 'Do you see that house by the side of the copse? That's Blackfaulds there, sir.'

Robert thanked him and continued. As he got closer to the house he wondered if the boy had been mistaken. He had expected something grander, more imposing. This looked more like a cottage or a gatehouse at the beginning of a large estate but, as he walked up to it, Robert could see that there was nothing beyond except the far edge of the loch and more open fields. It was a well-kept and respectable looking two-storey stone-built house. Sash and case windows were adorned with floral curtains and the porch at the front door was swept and neat. Before he could knock, he heard footsteps on the other side and realised someone must have spotted his approach.

A stout woman wearing an apron opened the door. She smoothed her pile of grey hair and smiled at him.

'Can I help you?' she asked, her accent more east coast than west.

'How do you do?' said Robert. 'I'm sorry to trouble you, but is this the home of Dr Sneddon?'

She nodded. 'I'm Mrs Sneddon. I'm afraid my husband is out at the moment, but he'll only be a short while. Do you have an appointment, Mr . . .?'

'Kinniburgh. I don't have an appointment. In point of fact, I'm enquiring about Euphemia McDougall.'

The woman smiled again, a little more thinly. She is wary as to my motives, Robert thought, and said breezily, 'I'm here on behalf of her parents, they have sent me to ask after her wellbeing.'

Mrs Sneddon's smile didn't falter but her expression remained guarded.

'I see. Please excuse me. My husband omitted to tell me you were due to visit.'

'I'm not sure if he knows. The arrangement was made at the last minute as I was due in Torrance on business anyway. Mrs McDougall's relatives merely asked me to ensure that she has settled in and is not in need of anything from home.'

Mrs Sneddon invited him in to wait in the parlour for the doctor's return.

Robert was surprised by how easily and effectively he had lied.

The heavy tick of a polished clock counted out the time as Robert sat at the parlour table, his finger tracing a pattern of embroidered flowers on the tablecloth. This floral theme was echoed in the curtains he had seen from outside, the wally tiles around the fireplace and some sprigs of rowan that were past their best but soldiered on in an earthenware vase in the middle of the table.

There was a sound of a door opening and closing and then some muttering before Dr Sneddon came into the room. Small and stout and grey, he and his wife made a matching pair. The doctor, however, was much more effusive and welcoming than his spouse or, perhaps, Robert thought, he had been hurriedly coached beforehand.

'You're here to enquire about Mrs McDougall, then?' Dr Sneddon asked. 'What can I tell you about her, Mr Kinniburgh? Do you wish to see her?'

'Only if you would recommend it, doctor. I don't know the lady myself and I wouldn't want to do anything that might upset her.'

'Quite so, sir. It is important that she is not unduly disturbed. However, she has been faring a great deal better since she arrived here. We are keen that this should be a home from home for her and company is not necessarily a bad thing, in my opinion. My wife is attending to her now and can let us know how she's keeping. All being well, I don't see why we shouldn't ask her downstairs to join us for a short while.'

'Thank you. I'm sure Mr and Mrs Rintoul would be happy to hear that I have been able to meet with their daughter.'

Robert told the doctor that he was a teacher at the Deaf and Dumb Institution and, as they waited, the doctor asked him about his work. Robert was mightily relieved that the doctor didn't seem to be curious about what business had brought him to the neighbourhood and allowed him to call in at Blackfaulds House. Perhaps his wife had forgotten to pass on that part of Robert's story. Soon, they had moved on to Robert's upbringing in nearby Kirkintilloch and

Robert was content to let the doctor expound on the changes to his hometown over the last few years, and how the plans for a railway link between Glasgow and Edinburgh might further affect the area.

Eventually, Mrs Sneddon returned and reported that Euphemia had got up from bed and would be delighted to join them. The doctor's wife excused herself and, when she came back some minutes later, brought with her tea, oatcakes and Mrs McDougall herself.

Euphemia McDougall was extraordinarily thin. Robert wasn't sure what he had been expecting but this fragile, almost brittle woman wasn't it. She was the kind of person that one would walk past in the street without a second glance. Unremarkable. Robert couldn't imagine her capable of violence, certainly not of the kind she had enacted on Jean and her dead baby.

Robert stood up as she entered the room alongside Mrs Sneddon. As the doctor's wife laid out a teapot, cups and saucers from a tray, Euphemia sat down in the chair to his right and clasped her hands together on her lap. She did not look at him but stared straight ahead at Dr Sneddon. She seemed to be concentrating very hard, as if the doctor was giving a lecture on a particularly complicated subject when, in fact, he was sitting silently as his wife poured their tea.

Once their tastes as to milk and sugar had been established and they were all furnished with a cup, Mrs Sneddon retreated to an armchair by the window, something Robert thought a little odd, there being a spare chair at the table.

There was no conversation as all of this occurred and the Sneddons did not introduce their guest to the patient, so Robert took the initiative and asked Euphemia how she was keeping.

'I'm very well, thank you,' she replied.

'Your father asked me to pass on his best wishes,' Robert continued. 'He has taken over responsibility for your care from your husband. He asked me to check that you are comfortable here.'

'My father?' Euphemia said, in a vague tone, as if she were unsure who exactly Robert was talking about.

She picked at the skin around her fingernails. Robert wondered at the disconnect between her outward appearance and these behavioural tics that hinted at some kind of turmoil under her calm appearance. He wished that he could speak to Euphemia without the presence of the Sneddons but felt he lacked the authority to make demands.

Instead, he asked, 'Mrs McDougall, are you content to remain here? Do you feel it aids your recovery?'

Euphemia nodded. 'I am quite well now,' she replied.

'Are you happy with Mrs McDougall's progress?' he asked Dr Sneddon.

'In so far as she is more rested than when she arrived here, then, yes, I feel she is on the road to recovery. However, it is only the start of a long road, Mr Kinniburgh. I would like to see her less dependent on medication to calm her nerves and aid her sleep. Hopefully, with time, we can affect a complete rest cure.'

'Does she speak of her home and her husband at all?' asked Robert.

Dr Sneddon shook his head. 'We don't encourage it. On arrival she was distressed about the life she had left behind, so we try to move her mind onto other things.'

'You don't recommend that patients talk about their difficulties?'

'No. We encourage stability and routine. A good night's sleep, a nutritious diet and useful occupation are more effective to give the heart ease, in my opinion.'

'I can understand that,' Robert said. 'I have no wish to distress Mrs McDougall further.'

Robert realised that he had assumed that Hector Rintoul's taking over payment of the fees to the Sneddons was due to paternal concern for his daughter, but now began to question this hypothesis. If Rintoul had really been worried, he would have made this journey himself. Perhaps Hector Rintoul was as happy to keep Euphemia away from society as Charles McDougall was? Robert found himself feeling sorry for this woman, whose nearest relatives found inconvenient at best and a threat to their liberty at worst.

They sipped their tea and chatted about the month's changeable weather. Mrs Sneddon showed Robert a piece of needlework that Euphemia had been working on. One of a set of antimacassars for the armchairs in the front room of the house. Euphemia yawned and Mrs Sneddon suggested that she have a nap before supper. Euphemia got up from the table and reached out her hand.

'Thank you for coming to visit me,' she said. 'It was a great pleasure to meet you.'

As she shook his hand her sleeve bunched up and Robert saw old welts of puckered scars that lined her wrist and travelled along the flesh of her inner arm.

57

~ Saturday, 22 March 1817:
The City Hospital and Poorhouse, Glasgow ~

The city's hospital and poorhouse was situated next to
Lawrie's Wood Yard on Great Clyde Street. Angus
Buchanan was familiar with the workings of the place,
having visited the building often, either on behalf of his
parishioners or in attendance at some fundraising event or
charitable meeting. He had even served on the board of
directors at one time as representative for his parish, alongside town councillors, merchants and tradesmen.

The poorhouse had been founded almost a century ago.
Its intention had been to care for destitute men, widows
and orphans of the city. The original H-shaped layout had
been much admired at the time of its construction for its
airiness and subsequent health-giving properties, but chronic
overcrowding – almost from the outset – had resulted in a
long list of deficiencies and calls for a new facility to be
provided. The problems were legion. There was little room
to separate the sick from the able-bodied; bathing facilities
were wholly inadequate with sometimes hundreds of inmates
taking their weekly bath in only one or two tubs; and the
addition of an infirmary to the rear of the building had
resulted in a lack of open-air exercise space.

Angus knew John Hardie, the superintendent, fairly well
and had been happy to take his word that no boy by the
name of Alexander or Sandy Campbell had been deposited
at the poorhouse in the days immediately following Jean's

arrest. However, if the last few weeks had taught Angus anything, it was that even an apparent truth was always worth testing. For this reason, Angus had agreed with Robert that it would be prudent to return to the poorhouse and double check the veracity of what the superintendent had relayed to him.

An orderly met him at the door and, as a well-kent face, Angus was permitted to make his own way up to the second storey of the building and along a white-washed corridor to the superintendent's office. The only thing accompanying him was an unpleasant smell; a mixture of stale boiled vegetables and bodily excretions. Now, he stood at the entrance of an empty office, having established that there was no sign of anyone around who could help him. Angus lingered for a moment, considering whether to return to the entranceway and enquire as to where else the superintendent might be.

Presently, a figure came along the corridor towards him. Angus recognised the bounding gait of the superintendent.

'Angus, are you looking for me?' Hardie called out as he approached.

'I was, but I've found you now, so all's well.'

Hardie's shirtsleeves were pushed up above the elbow and he began to roll them down.

'I was in the basement,' he said by way of explanation. 'We've had another flood, what with all this rain. The river's running so fast, it's a bugger trying to shore anything up against it.'

'Och, that's a pity,' said Angus. 'It must be a worry for you.'

John Hardie shook his head, ruefully. 'Happens all the time. The defences at the waterfront are non-existent. I'm sick of telling the trustees about it. The whole bloody lot of us will just float down the river one of these days. We'll end up in Greenock, so we will. Anyway, what can I do for you?'

'Do you remember a few weeks ago, I came looking for a young lad that I thought might have been brought to you?' asked Angus.

'Aye, from the police office. Cameron or something – wasn't it?'

'Campbell,' said Angus, 'Sandy Campbell. He's the son of one of my parishioners.'

'Aye, of course I remember, but we didn't have anyone of that name here.'

Angus nodded. 'I know, but I was wondering if he might have been put here under another name. Is that possible?'

'Anything's possible, Angus. What age did you say this lad was?'

'Six years old.'

'Come on down to the receiving room,' said Hardie. 'We'll check in the ledger.'

'Thank you, John. I know you're busy, and I appreciate it. I might be on a hiding to nothing, but I need to make sure.'

Hardie showed Angus to a door at the back of his office and the two men took a set of back stairs down to the ground floor, where another long corridor presented itself. The old stone walls had been whitewashed at some point but much of the colour had faded or chipped. The exposed red sandstone made a pattern of sorts. A series of wooden doors punctuated the corridor, most of them open, as it was the middle of the day. As Angus walked alongside the superintendent, he caught glimpses of groups of people engaged in laundering clothes and preparing vegetables. They passed by a bare schoolroom where children sat in rows and bowed their heads over their work.

When they reached the receiving room, Hardie ushered Angus through a large waiting area and into an antechamber that had a desk and chair and a cabinet filled with books and papers.

Hardie opened the cabinet and took out a large foolscap ledger. Its leather binding was worn and discoloured in places through almost constant use. He located a broad bookmark of faded yellow ribbon and lifted the pages aside to show the most recent entries. Each page held the hand-written details of an inmate, with their surname repeated and inscribed in larger, bolder letters in the outside top corner of the page. Angus had been present when new inmates were accepted into the poorhouse and had some-times answered on behalf of those who were unable, for whatever reason, to provide the circumstances of their lives and how they had arrived in this place. From memory, he knew there were questions on personal details and causes of infirmity, as well as a list of dwelling places in order to determine which parish council should pay for the upkeep of the inmate.

Hardie skimmed the text before him and asked, 'What date did you say the boy might have been brought here?'

'No earlier than February the twenty-fourth,' Angus replied.

'I'll go back and see if any boys of that approximate age have been brought in,' said Hardie.

Hardie looked at a number of pages, shaking his head when he located the age of the inmate.

'Hold on,' he said, 'this one's for a boy aged five. Does any of this ring a bell, Angus?'

Angus peered at the page and tried to decipher the unfamiliar handwriting. It was neatly done, and the infor-mation was well laid out, but it took him a while to fathom some abbreviations and official terminology. What struck him was that the surname in the outer corner of the page was Wilson.

'This boy is called Alexander Wilson, is that right?'

'Yes, it would appear so. I don't remember the wee boy being brought in,' said Hardie. 'That's my deputy's signature at the bottom. Hold on, I'll send for him.'

Superintendent Hardie opened the door to his office and called out to a boy in the corridor.

'Away and fetch Mr Ingram, Billy. Shift yourself, son, it's important.'

A few minutes later, Angus and Hardie were joined by Michael Ingram, a short, portly man wearing plaid trousers and a heavy shirt with a drawstring at the collar. Hardie beckoned him in and, eschewing preliminaries, questioned the man about the admission.

'See this wee boy, name of Wilson, what do you remember about his being brought in?'

Ingram scanned the entry in the ledger and dredged his memory for a moment.

'He had been found, alone, at the docks in Partick. He seemed to have been abandoned. When I asked him about his parents, he got very distressed. He kept saying his mother had been taken away, which I took to mean she was either in the jail, the madhouse or dead. I couldn't get him to tell me any more than that.'

Although there was no list of previous addresses for this Alexander Wilson, Angus noticed that it had been recorded that he had brown eyes and blond hair.

'The physical description noted here sounds very like the boy that I'm looking for. And he said this was his name?' Angus asked.

'He knew his name was Alexander. He didn't understand what we wanted when we asked him about his surname. We gave him Wilson because that's the name of the gentleman who brought him here.'

'Really?' Angus asked. 'Did you know the man, Michael?'

'Yes. Cunningham Wilson.'

Angus looked at the superintendent in surprise. 'The doctor that has a practice on the Dumbarton Road?'

'Aye, that's right,' said Hardie.

58

~ Saturday, 22 March 1817:
Candleriggs, Glasgow ~

Charles McDougall would rather have been anywhere in the world than in Hector Rintoul's office. However, needs must, and he was in want of money. Without ready cash, it was proving difficult to keep the various strands of his life from strangling him by degrees. After Euphemia had been removed, he had wasted no time in shutting up the house in Partickhill and dismissing that inconvenient maid, Martha Sproull.

Charles had packed up a few clothes and decamped to a small room above the shipyard at the docks. He would have to find a buyer for the house eventually, but he thought it prudent to lay low for as long as possible.

He had hoped that Jean Campbell would have been found guilty and hanged by now. That outcome, coupled with Euphemia's relocation to the asylum, should have presented him with a long-overdue clean sheet on which he might begin a new chapter of his life.

It was not to be. Just as he was congratulating himself for cleaning up the mess caused by a mad wife and a deaf hoor, he learnt that the jury had judged the case not proven. He had had to wait until the next day to read an account of the case in the newspaper, and that didn't tell him a great deal.

Charles assumed that the bleeding-heart teacher and the do-gooder minister had succeeded in making the jury feel sorry for Jean Campbell. It was a relief, however, to read that the teacher, Kinniburgh, had been entrusted by the authorities to take the bitch back to her own people. The sooner she was away from Glasgow, in Charles's view, the better.

The financial outlay involved, both in keeping Euphemia quiet, and his business afloat, was crippling him. Charles hoped to persuade Rintoul to bridge the gap in his cashflow. So, here he was, begging bowl in hand, forced to crawl to his patronising father-in-law, who had plenty of money but only because it had been passed down to him from his wealthy family. It sickened Charles that this man could lord it over him purely because of an accident of birth.

The door opposite opened and Hector regarded his son-in-law over the rims of his pince-nez spectacles. Charles was convinced that the glasses and the gesture were deliberate affectations – adopted to bolster Hector's view of himself as a refined and educated man who never got his hands dirty.

'Charles. Do come through.' Hector held the door open for his visitor, an act that, paradoxically, felt intimidating rather than subservient.

Charles stood awkwardly in the centre of the room as Hector prowled around the perimeter, taking an inordinate amount of time to get to his own chair before attending to the comfort of his guest.

'Sit down, won't you?' Hector said.

Hector Rintoul was as neat and manicured as a well-kept garden border. His clothes were starched and freshly laundered and his fine grey hair cut precisely at the nape of his neck, just above his necktie. Nothing merged or overlapped with Hector. Every aspect of his appearance was as tabulated as the balance sheets he worked with daily.

'I'm glad we've got this opportunity to have a chat,' Hector began, that last word spat out sarcastically, his lips pursing as if he were choosing between smiling and snarling at Charles. 'I've made arrangements to take over the long-term responsibility for the care of Euphemia. Her keep is paid until the end of this week, but I've told the Sneddons that I'll take on the burden from there.'

Charles furrowed his brow. This wasn't what he had been expecting at all. He had primed himself to act the concerned husband, full of regrets at not being able to give his wife the care and comfort that she deserved in her present difficulties. He ought to be happy that the performance wouldn't be necessary, and that Hector had already solved one of his current problems, but he couldn't help feeling that a rug had been pulled from under him. Since when did Euphemia's father do anything without being grovelled to first?

'That's very kind of you, Hector,' Charles said tentatively. 'I had been hoping to talk to you about how to ensure Euphemia is taken care of. This whole business has kept me from my duties at the shipyard and I could do with some breathing space to get things financially buoyant again.'

'Yes,' said Hector, 'I was disappointed to see that the last two repayments on your loan haven't been made. That's a fair amount of time passed and I've still to see some return on my investment.'

'Aye, well,' Charles muttered, 'there was a great deal of outlay at the beginning and I'm chasing up my own creditors at the moment. With all this carry-on of Euphemia's, I've had more immediate problems to deal with.'

Hector took off his spectacles and began cleaning them with a handkerchief. 'I see. You should consider taking someone on to do your administration. It doesn't do to let things slip. No matter the provocation,' he said, pointedly.

Charles didn't reply.

Hector replaced his spectacles and began folding the handkerchief. 'Anyway, I hear you've shut up the house.'

How the fuck does he know that? thought Charles. I only did it a fortnight ago. This bastard has his fingers all over my business.

Charles tried not to betray his annoyance. 'Temporarily. I didn't think it was worth paying the ser-vants to keep it running when I'm hardly there.'

'And now you're staying above the shop, so to speak?' Hector gave him a sideways glance and looked like he'd stepped in some dog shite.

'As I said, it's a temporary arrangement.'

Hector leant forward over a huge pad of blotting paper in from of him.

'Let's cut to the chase, Charles. When you married my daughter, I invested heavily in both your domestic and professional life. That was over five years ago. I would have hoped that, by now at the very least, I would be seeing a return on that investment. I also had some expectation that you would be doing your duty as a husband. It's a pity that the match hasn't produced any issue. Regardless, I'd have hoped that you would have been ensuring that my daughter's welfare is paramount.'

Charles could feel his bile rising.

'Look. Don't take me for a fool, Hector. You passed your lunatic offspring on to me. Her passage was bought with your money. Then you left me to mop up the mess.'

'I'll thank you to temper your language when you talk about my daughter,' Hector snarled. 'Euphemia has always been fragile. She has suffered with her nerves from a young age, but she was no lunatic. If she's descended into madness, I can only assume that you helped her get there.'

'Living with that bitch,' Charles yelled, 'I'm surprised it's not me that's in that fucking place!'

319

Hector Rintoul wasn't a man to get into a shouting match, especially not with someone as coarse as he considered Charles McDougall to be. He studied his son-in-law carefully and took his time, and a breath, before responding.

'I will not discuss Euphemia with you any longer. I will take care of her and you will leave her alone.'

'I'm her husband, you stupid old fool. I'll be the judge of what happens to her.'

'You'll sign over guardianship of Euphemia. This very day.'

'Really?' Charles laughed.

Hector smiled. 'If you want me to pay the Sneddons, you will.'

That stopped Charles in his tracks. Silence hung between them for a few moments.

Charles considered the situation for a moment.

'If you want to play that game,' he said, 'give me the papers and I'll sign her over to you. Good fucking riddance. She's yours for the duration, mind, don't be trying to foist her back on to me if, by some miracle, she ever gets out of that madhouse.'

'Well, that's one issue dealt with,' Hector said. 'What about the house and your business loan? That house was paid for by me.'

'It was a wedding gift,' said Charles, incredulously.

'But I still own it, Charles. According to the documents we had drawn up. You do remember the documents we drew up, don't you?'

Charles's face was like thunder. 'You bought it for your daughter.'

'She doesn't need it anymore and I want my money back on that business loan. I doubt you'll be able to raise much from your shipyard.'

'Take the fucking house, then,' Charles raged at him. 'You're not getting your hands on my yard.'

'I wouldn't want your yard,' Hector said. 'By all accounts, you're not even breaking even. Good luck paying your men without any more money from me and good luck getting contracts once I whisper in the right ears.'

59

They came at him not two minutes after he left Rintoul's office.

Charles stepped out onto Candleriggs, still fuming at the way he had been treated by Hector. There were a few other people walking along the street and some others hanging around doorways and close mouths.

Suddenly, a man walked right in front of him, tripping him up.

'Watch where you're going,' he shouted at the fellow, who rather took the wind out of Charles's sails by being full of apologies.

The man was poor-looking and wore only shirtsleeves, though these were topped with a collared fawn waistcoat and Charles could see a watch chain hanging from a pocket. An ill-fitting bowler hat perched atop a mop of dark red hair. He had a slight Irish accent but didn't mumble incoherently like most of the other taigs Charles had come across. He helped Charles up and patted him down and Charles thanked him cautiously, relieved that no real harm had been done.

By this time, another man had approached them and was hovering around, perhaps anticipating that a fight was about to ensue. However, Charles had no wish to linger, and he straightened his clothes, gave a cursory nod of acknowledgement and hurried south, making for the Trongate, where he had an appointment with a large whisky. As usual, his dealings with his father-in-law had left a bad taste in his mouth that needed to be expunged.

He jumped as he felt an arm around his shoulder and saw again the red-haired man who had caused him to trip over. Charles took an instinctive inventory of his money and pocket watch, noting their location in case the man had decided he might be an easy mark.

The red-haired man just winked at him. 'Can I have a word, captain?' he said jovially, and steered Charles into the opening of a close.

It was narrow and damp and smelt of decay. A good number of carts had been upended and stacked against the wall on one side. On the other, Charles caught glimpses of people retreating inside stairwells, like tortoises into shells. It was bizarrely quiet away from the bustle of the street.

Another heavy hand on his back, his arm twisted behind him and his bones cracked like gunshot. Before he could process what was happening, he was slammed head-first into the brickwork opposite him and he blacked out.

∼

It was so dark in the cramped confines of the close that, when Charles came to, he couldn't tell how much time had passed. It could have been a few minutes or a few hours. Blood and phlegm had gathered in his throat and he gagged on it, howking it up in a panic lest it choke him, spraying the mess of it over his chest.

He could hardly fathom the pain that was concentrated at the bridge of his nose and spread outwards across his face. It was clamped around his head like a vice. He couldn't bear to move, to blink even, the curl of his eyelids like steel clamps on his eyeballs.

The close was empty apart from the two men who had accosted him. The red-haired one in the bowler hat, who had tripped him up and called him captain, was sitting on an upturned crate, leaning back against the wall and smoking a pipe as if nothing in the world was more natural.

The other one, a well-built labourer with a shock of thick dark hair, was standing a few feet away, staring at Charles but saying nothing.

Charles tried to suppress the fear that was mounting in his gut and began to take in the geography of his surroundings more carefully. He could see the narrow entrance to the close about twenty feet in front of him. He knew that beyond that was Candleriggs. The brick outbuilding that he had been driven into was some kind of store or coal hole maybe. To his left was a set of rackety steps leading upwards, to what he didn't know.

This area of Glasgow lay between the crush of the Saltmarket and the uniformity of George Street. The front that Candleriggs presented to the street was fairly respectable but, behind the polished doorways leading to offices and the orderly windows of shops, lay a maze of closes, vennels, workshops and store yards.

There were still plenty of thatched roofs and wooden staircases from medieval times, cheek by jowl against hurriedly thrown-up stone tenements that had become unbearably overcrowded no sooner than they were erected. It was a warren full of the worst of humanity where no one would want to end up, under any circumstances, far less those that Charles found himself in.

He tried to shift himself into an upright sitting position. Perhaps if he offered these men the money he had on him, they would let him go. But, if they wanted money, wouldn't they have emptied his pockets and taken off with it already? Why were they sitting here still? What the hell were they waiting for?

The dark-haired man fished a bottle out of his jacket pocket and took a drink. He coughed as the spirit went down. He wiped the neck of the bottle on his sleeve and then handed it over to his partner. He recommenced his scrutiny of Charles.

'Not so brave now, are you?' he said.

Charles's stared at him, trying to work out if he knew this man. He looked vaguely familiar, and he thought he might have seen him somewhere before. But then, they all looked the same, these taigs. Dirty and uncouth. This one had dark hair that fell over his eyes and patches of his fair skin were sunburnt between dark eyes and straggly beard. He slowly divested himself of his jacket, hanging it over a corner of one of the upturned carts. He unhooked his braces from his shoulders and pulled his shirt over his head. The hair on his chest was as dark as that on top of his head. It spread down his stomach and disappeared into the waistband of his trousers.

Charles's voice was thick with fear. When he spoke the blood left in his throat moved up into his mouth and his voice sounded strangulated and hoarse. 'Is it money you want?' he asked. 'I can give you money.'

'Don't you worry, captain, we'll take your money,' the bare-chested man smiled at him almost benignly, 'but this isn't going to be a painless transaction. I thought you would have got that message already.'

The red-haired man drank from the bottle and laughed. His previous obsequious demeanour had completely melted away and Charles thought he had the measure of them both now. Ignorant navvies out looking for a fight.

Then the dark-haired one said something that turned even that theory on its head.

'My name's Jim Donnelly,' he said steadily. 'I'm here for Jean Campbell, Mr McDougall.'

With that, Charles fell silent, and the two Irishmen walked towards him. Jim Donnelly reached down and dragged him upwards. Leant his forearm on Charles's neck and pinned him to the wall.

There was a look of grim relish on the taig's face. As if he had hungered for this moment. Charles shut his eyes and did something he'd not done for years. He began to pray.

60

∼ Sunday, 23 March 1817:
The Broomielaw, Glasgow ∼

There were quite a number of people on the quay that afternoon despite the incessant rain and a cold east wind. The north bank of the river was a busy place where cargoes of all kinds were delivered and collected.

Only a few were there to catch the boat that took passengers out of the city to Port Glasgow, where they could make onward connections to the west coast and the islands.

Robert and Angus stood to one side, Robert checking the tickets that Angus had bought with Succoth's money and Angus holding a battered umbrella over them both.

Jean and Sandy sat on top of a pile of flour sacks that had been in the middle of the forecourt. They seemed oblivious to the rain, enthralled by each other's company. Jean occasionally peered down at her son as if he had been returned to her by a host of angels rather than a commonplace Glaswegian cleric. At her feet she kept a small bag made up of a few of her belongings and supplemented with clothes and other necessary items gifted to her and Sandy by the Buchanans and various members of their congregation.

The boat had arrived yesterday evening, and its rested crew were busy loading mail and bags of supplies to be disseminated at Port Glasgow. Passengers were the last to get on board.

A cry went up from the street as a middle-aged woman held her skirts up and ran to the dock. Jean was oblivious as the woman pushed her way through the throng of people moving towards the gangplank, but Sandy looked round and tugged urgently at his mother's sleeve.

The boy tapped frantically at his chin with his index and middle finger.

It's my auntie. It's my auntie. Look!

Jean turned around and saw Aunt Nancy rushing toward her. The older woman stumbled on the wet slabs and Robert and Jean reached out to grab her.

The two women embraced, blocking the queue. Angus ushered them out of the way of the other people and Robert took hold of Sandy's hand.

They formed a knot beside the boat and Aunt Nancy first held Jean's head in her hands and then bent down to Sandy and kissed his head over and over again.

She clenched her fist and pushed it in a circle against her breastbone. *I'm sorry. I'm so sorry for all your trouble.*

Jean smiled. She clasped both of her thumbs and index fingers together and drew them outwards from her, as if she were conducting a particularly energetic orchestra. *Don't worry. You did what you could for us.*

The two women held each other for a long time and then broke apart. Aunt Nancy reached into her skirts and brought out a felt bag, tied together with ribbon. Jean opened it. Inside was a pock-marked tin thimble with threads, needles and pins. Aunt Nancy gave Sandy a poke of roasted nuts to take on the boat and kissed him again.

Robert was sorry to break them up, but he had to make sure Jean got home safely. The women said their goodbyes and Jean, Sandy and Robert boarded the boat.

61

~ Wednesday, 26 March 1817:
Islay, the Inner Hebrides ~

They stood, awkwardly, on the quay, both of them looking inland towards a string of one-storey cottages.

On the beach, a group of children played, running barefoot along the shore, dodging the waves as they spread over the sand. A lone heron, hunched in on itself, perched on a rocky outcrop that peeked above the sea. Fishermen's boats, some freshly painted, some that had seen better days, lay tied up and waiting for their masters in the shallows.

Alec Campbell traversed the pier. He seemed to know most of the islanders who were getting ready to travel on the boat or who were waiting to load or unload goods. Jean's father was dressed in tweed breeches, stout boots and wool waistcoat. His only concession to the day's surprisingly warm weather was the leaving of his jacket with the horse and cart.

The boat for the mainland waited patiently for the hour of its departure, bobbing gently on the calm expanse of water that hugged the island's coastline.

Robert was in two minds about leaving. It was like inhabiting the body of a fragile Colossus, one who had one foot lingering on Islay and the other poised, ready to leap over the sound and run home to Margaret, to the children and the school, to the new baby who would shortly be on its way.

This pull in two directions confused him. What was it that he couldn't bear to let go? Not Jean herself. Well, not as a woman, as someone he craved a romantic attachment to, no matter what Margaret suggested. It was the solving of the puzzle he would miss. The resolution of Jean's case was not to his liking, in terms of it being fundamentally unjust. No one had been brought to book for the killing of Jean's baby. Euphemia McDougall had been shut away in an asylum, controlled and contained to the last. And Charles McDougall, complicit and evasive, had not been damaged by the case. Or, at least, not on the surface.

Robert wondered whether, underneath the bombastic exterior that he presented to the world, Charles McDougall's crimes were eating him up from the inside. Shame was a powerful engine. Just as some human beings strove to do good, to improve their lot and that of those less fortunate than themselves, so others strove to hide their inadequacies, their faults and occasionally the evil that they visited on others. It seemed to Robert that Charles McDougall was consumed by shame. Shame about his origins, shame about his business dealings, shame about the way he had treated his wife and the hatred he bore towards her.

Why am I thinking about this again? he asked himself. Some things are destined to remain hidden. This problem, the one that had festered and mutated in the house at Partickhill, was not one that he could solve.

A boatman gave a signal and the crowd unravelled; those that were staying held back and those that were going picked up their luggage and made their way to the gangplank. Robert hoisted his bag onto one shoulder and tucked the ends of his scarf inside his jacket.

'Goodbye, Alec. Thank you for your hospitality.'

Alec Campbell shook Robert's hand.

'You're welcome anytime, son. Thank you for bringing our lass back safely.'

Jean stepped forward. *I don't how to thank you. If you hadn't come to the prison, they would have hanged me.*

Perhaps. Robert stuck out his thumb and pinkie and jiggled his right hand. *There is no need to thank me, I was glad to do it.*

You will be a father soon, she said, rubbing her forefinger and thumb together.

Robert nodded. *In August, God willing.*

Jean studied him for a moment. She reached out and brought her hand to his face and cupped her palm on his cheek. Then she touched her own cheek and lifted her palm from it into the space between them.

The clean-shaven one.

~ *Author's Note* ~

In 1817, the real Robert Kinniburgh interpreted Jean Campbell's plea as she stood trial for murder at the High Court in Edinburgh. *Hear No Evil* is a largely fictional account of the lead up to the crime, the trial, and its aftermath. Some characters are loosely based on real people, while others are entirely fictitious.

I first heard of Jean Campbell's case when I was working at Deaf Connections in Glasgow, from historian and author, Robert J Smith, whose book, *The City Silent*, includes a brief account of the trial and its significance to the history of the Deaf community. I followed that trail to the National Records of Scotland, hoping to find out more about Jean Campbell's experience of being a Deaf woman in the early nineteenth century. Frustratingly, beyond some cursory facts about her life, Jean is essentially absent from the official records, so I decided to invent her story.

The building that was Edinburgh's Deaf and Dumb Institution still exists today in Chessels Court, just off the Canongate. Kinniburgh took over the running of the school from Thomas Braidwood, who was influential in the development of British Sign Language (BSL). In the early nineteenth century, there were no widespread signed languages in the way we understand them today.

Much of the contemporary reporting around Jean Campbell's case treats signing as an anomaly, something weird and freakish to entertain a readership or to be analysed by academics. For a modern audience, these attitudes seem antiquated and discriminatory. However, it is worth remembering that BSL was only officially recognised as a language by the UK Government in 2003. There is still a long way to go to achieve meaningful equality.

~ *Acknowledgements* ~

Thanks to all my Deaf friends for sharing your experiences with me. I hope you enjoy the book and feel I've done your community justice.

Much of my research was guided by Deaf History Scotland, a charity that conserves Deaf heritage for future generations. Several people were incredibly generous with their time and expertise. Dr Lilian Lawson gave me feedback on my portrayal of Deaf characters. Dr Ella Leith shared her knowledge about the world Robert Kinniburgh inhabited and inspired me with her enthusiasm. Professor Claire McDiarmid, from the University of Strathclyde, answered my questions on the Scottish legal system. On Islay, Donald, Catriona, and Angus Bell, and the staff and volunteers at the Museum of Islay Life helped me to fill in Jean's backstory.

The friendship and support from staff and students on the MLitt in Creative Writing at the University of Glasgow meant the world to me. A New Writers Award from the Scottish Book Trust gave me time and space to get the book completed. Huge thanks to Dr Zoë Strachan, the best tutor and mentor I could have wished for. During the pandemic, it's been a joy to be part of the #VWG, whose good advice and humour kept me on track.

I'm so lucky to have the professionalism and encouragement of my agent, Jenny Hewson, and the lovely team at Lutyens and Rubinstein. I'm very grateful to my publisher,

Lisa Highton, and everyone at Two Roads Books for choosing my book and steering me through the publishing process.

Much love and thanks to my brilliant pals – Helen Fleming, Pat Leanord, Sharon Mackay, Paula Murdoch, Rachel McNeill, and Susan Cameron for chipping in ideas and chivvying me along.

I'm grateful to my fantastic daughters, Rosie and Juliet, and to my mum, Joan, for feedback on my early drafts. Lastly, I couldn't have done this without Peter, who kept paying the bills and believing in me.

∾ *About the Author* ∾

Sarah Smith is a writer from Glasgow whose work has been published in a variety of journals and anthologies, including *New Writing Scotland, 50GS, Flashback Fiction, Gilded Dirt* and *From Glasgow to Saturn*. In 2018, she completed an MLitt in Creative Writing from the University of Glasgow and went on to gain a Scottish Book Trust New Writers Award in 2019. She has experience of working with the Deaf community, including most recently at Deaf Connections in Glasgow, where she first came across the remarkable story of Jean Campbell and Robert Kinniburgh.